SPECTACULAR HAIR

A STEP-BY-STEP GUIDE TO 46 GORGEOUS STYLES

By
Eric Mayost

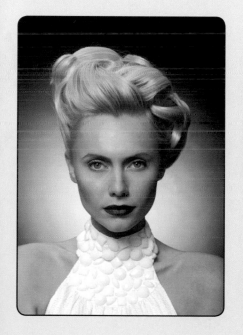
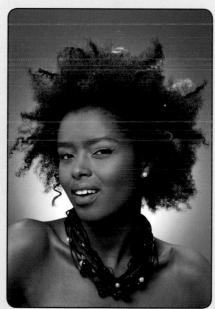
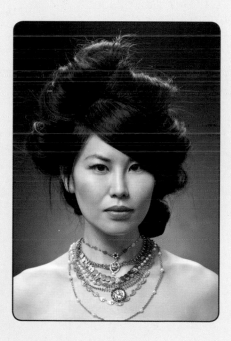

STERLING

New York / London
www.sterlingpublishing.com

Photography by Roee Fainburg

Design and layout by Ariane Rybski

Edited by Shoshana Brickman and Daniel Zilberberg

Styling by Avivit Lamdan

Makeup by Perry Ohaion

10 9 8 7 6 5 4 3 2 1

Published by Sterling Publishing
387 Park Avenue South, New York, NY 10016
© 2010 by Penn Publishing Ltd.
Distributed in Canada by Sterling Publishing
C/o Canadian Manda Group, 165 Dufferin Street
Toronto, Ontario, Canada M6K 3H6
Distributed in the United Kingdom by GMC Distribution Services
Castle Place, 166 High Street, Lewes, East Sussex, England BN7 1XU
Distributed in Australia by Capricorn Link (Australia) Pty. Ltd.
P.O. Box 704, Windsor, NSW 2756, Australia

Sterling ISBN 978-1-4027-6898-9

For information about custom editions, special sales, and premium and corporate purchases, please contact Sterling Special Sales at 800–805–5489 or specialsales@sterlingpublishing.com.

CONTENTS

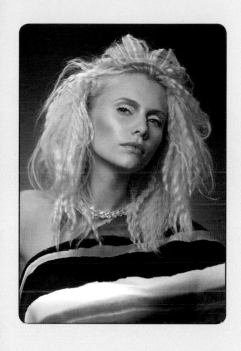

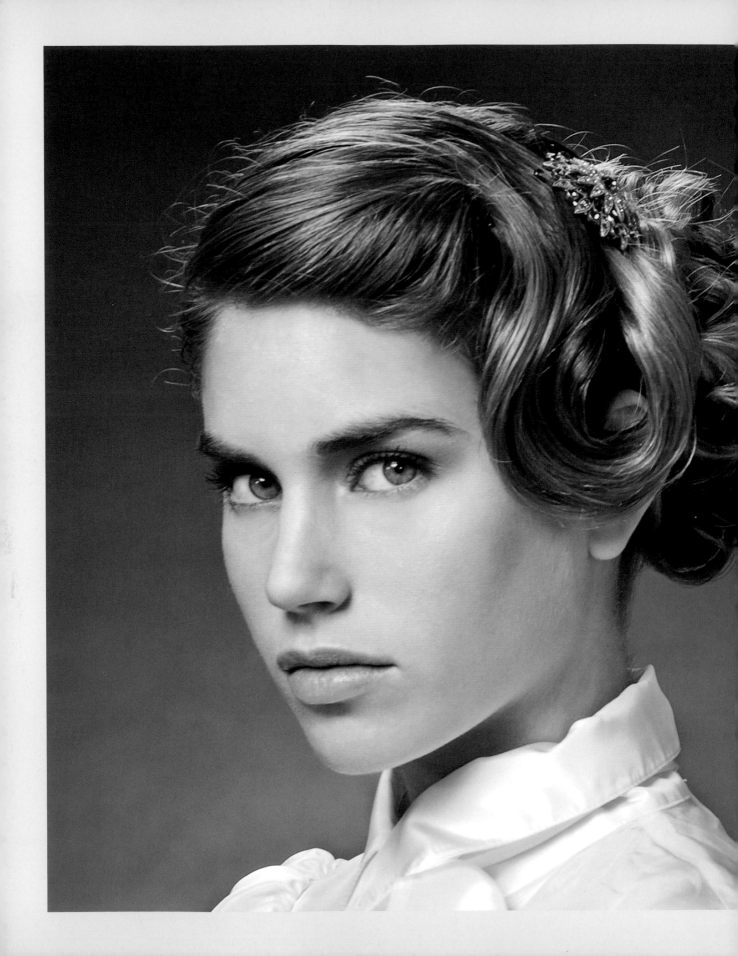

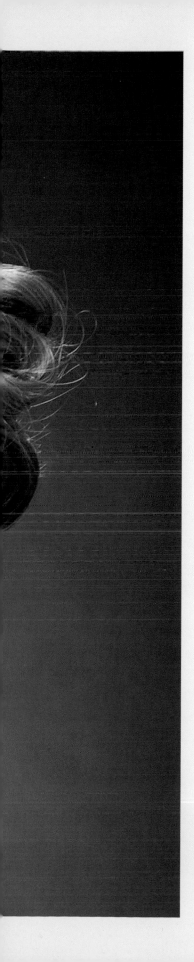

INTRODUCTION

Everyone wants great looking hair and a style that won't go unnoticed. But going to a hair salon every time you want an extra-special look is expensive and time-consuming. Instead of rearranging your day around a stylist's schedule, why not learn how to style your hair yourself? Not only will you save money and time; you'll also have the thrill of knowing you created your own fabulous hairstyle.

In **Spectacular Hair**, you'll find exceptional styles that are perfect for every event. Whether it's a prom or a movie, a wedding or a romantic walk, an evening at the ballet or a night of dancing at the hottest club in town, you'll find something to suit your style.

Every hairstyle in this book includes simple, step-by-step instructions and plenty of photographs. You'll learn how to create salon styles in the comfort of your own home. If some prove too tricky to handle yourself, invite a friend over and style each other's hair. Become an inspiration to others by setting a hairstyle standard of your own.

ABOUT THE AUTHOR:

Eric Mayost has been styling hair since he was nineteen years old and has worked with some of the world's leading hairstylists. In addition to hairstyling, he studied art and graphic design. Eric has designed hairstyles for cover shoots of some of the world's leading fashion magazines, and he carved a career for himself by giving stars the glamorous looks they desire. In this book, Eric shares with readers the valuable tools, techniques, and experience he has acquired.

Eric is one of the founders of solostyling.com, a "do-it-yourself" hairstyling website. He has been managing his successful hair salon since 2002, keeping himself and his staff at the forefront of hairstyling fashion.

ESSENTIAL SUPPLIES AND TIPS

To create your own fabulous hairstyles, you'll need a few basic supplies. You may have many of these items already. If not, they can be found in hair salons, beauty supply shops, and department stores. There is also a vast amount of equipment for sale online.

Blow dryer
Hair is often washed and blow dried before styling. In many cases, you'll also need a blow dryer for the styling process.

Bobby pins
These small pins are used to secure hair close to the head. A bobby pin is made of a single piece of wire, its two ends bent together. One side of the pin is straight and the other kinked.

Clips
Metal and plastic clips of various sizes are used to hold sections of hair while other sections are being styled.

Crimping iron
This is used to shape hair into crimps.

Curling iron
This is essential for making curls. Curling irons come in various sizes, so choose one that produces the type of curl you desire.

Diffuser
This adds volume and accentuates curly hair.

Elastic bands
These are used to secure ponytails and braids. Choose elastic bands that are gentle on the hair and don't rip it. Neutral colors are best, since some hairstyles reveal them.

Hair accessories
Hair bands, ribbons, jewelry and many other accessories are used in a number of hairstyles as decorations and finishing touches.

Hair extensions
These are natural or synthetic hair additions that are integrated into the hair to add volume or length. Hair extensions may be long or short, straight or curly, braided or left loose. You can choose one that either matches or contrasts with your natural hair color. Hair extensions can be used over and over again.

Hairnets
Use these to gather either hair extensions or natural hair.

Holding spray

Spray this onto your hair as you sculpt it, and spray again to hold the finished hairstyle in place. The holding spray you choose should preserve the style without making your hair too stiff.

Moisturizing cream

Apply the cream to curly hair or when curling straight hair to keep the hair from drying out.

Molding wax

The wax is applied to dry hair to add moisture. It also helps sculpt hair and achieve a strong hold.

Round brush

Also known as a radial brush, it is used to shape the hair while blow drying, and to add volume and body to dry hair.

Sponge

Sponges are integrated into hairstyles to add structure and volume. Match them to your hair color to conceal them beneath hair or hair extensions. To make your own sponges, wrap hair extensions in a transparent hairnet and shape as desired. Sponges can be used several times, so be sure to care for them properly.

Styling cream

Apply the cream generously to dry hair for a softer touch. It is especially important when blow drying, since heat can damage the hair.

Styling gel

This adds moisture to dry hair and helps hold the sculpted style in place.

Tail comb

Also called rattail combs, they have teeth at one end and a fine point at the other. Use the teeth for backcombing hair, and use the fine point for making a part to divide the hair into sections.

Wide-tooth comb

Use this to separate locks of hair.

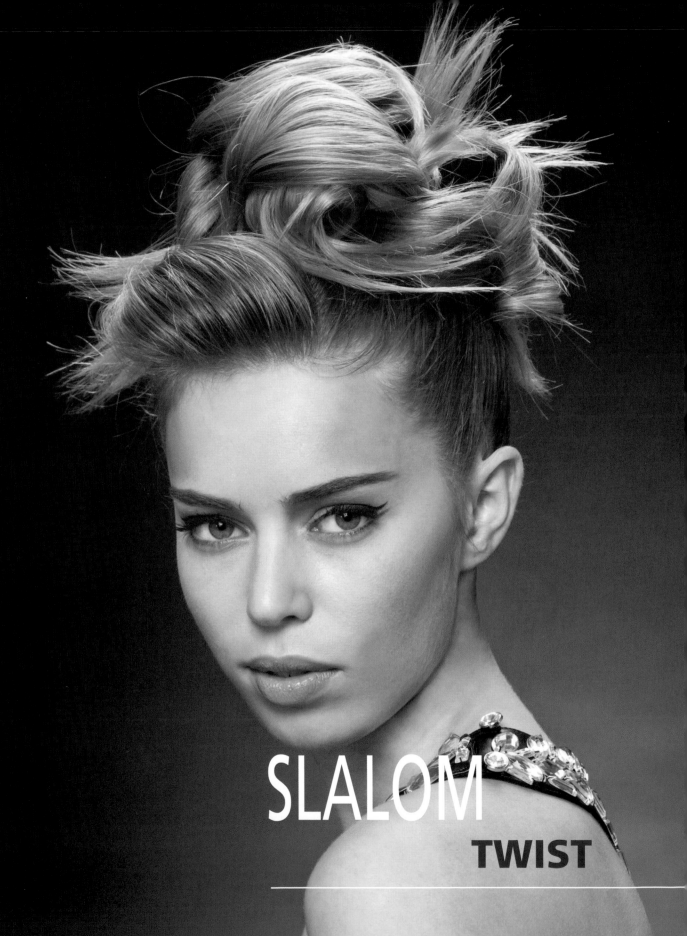

SLALOM

TWIST

1

This eclectic style is funky and fun. It features large and small loops of hair that are oriented in every direction to create a crafted yet chaotic look.

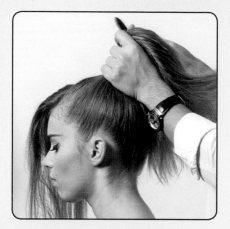

1

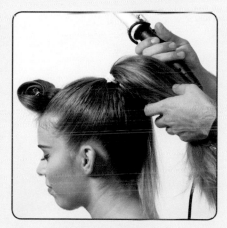

2

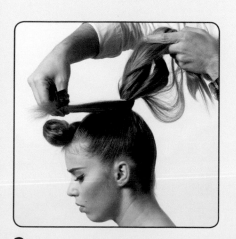

3

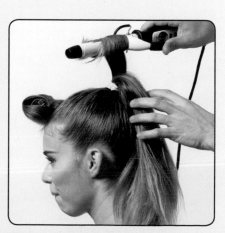

4

1. Wash and blow dry the hair. Separate the bangs from the rest of the hair; then gather the hair in a high ponytail.

2. Secure the ponytail with an elastic band and secure the bangs with a clip.

3. Curl a 1-inch section of hair in the ponytail with a medium curling iron.

4. Hold the curling iron to secure the curl; then mist with holding spray.

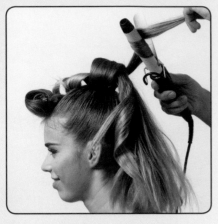

5

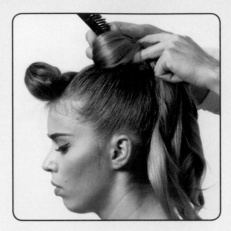

6

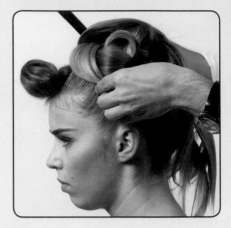

7

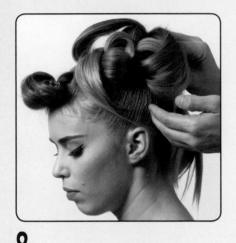

8

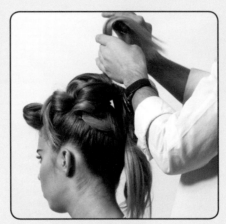

9

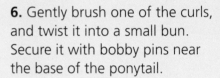

5. Repeat the process, section by section, to curl the entire ponytail.

6. Gently brush one of the curls, and twist it into a small bun. Secure it with bobby pins near the base of the ponytail.

7. Gently brush out another lock, and twist it into a bun that wraps over the first bun. Pin it to the head with a bobby pin.

8. Repeat the process to secure several curled locks of hair near the base of the ponytail. Try to make each curl a different size, or orient them in different directions.

9. Secure some of the locks above the first set of curls, to add height.

10. Adjust the arrangement of the locks, so that the curls are asymmetrical and the hairstyle looks different from every angle.

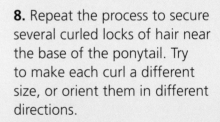

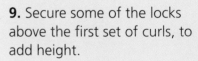

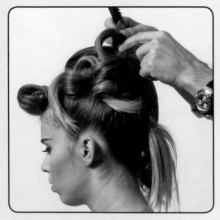

10

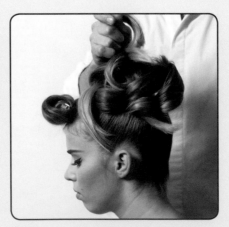

11

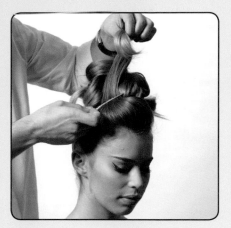

12

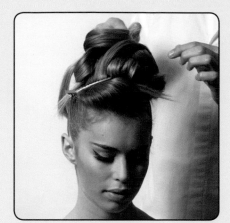

13

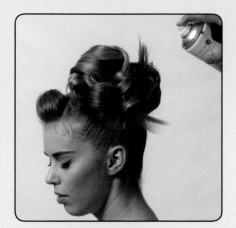

14

11. When you are satisfied with the arrangement, secure the hairstyle with more bobby pins, and mist with holding spray.

12. Comb the bangs backward, and make a loose fold at the front, to create height. Secure the bangs temporary with a clip.

13. Tuck the ends of the bangs into the collection of curls at the top of the head.

14. Secure the hairstyle with extra bobby pins, as required, and mist with holding spray.

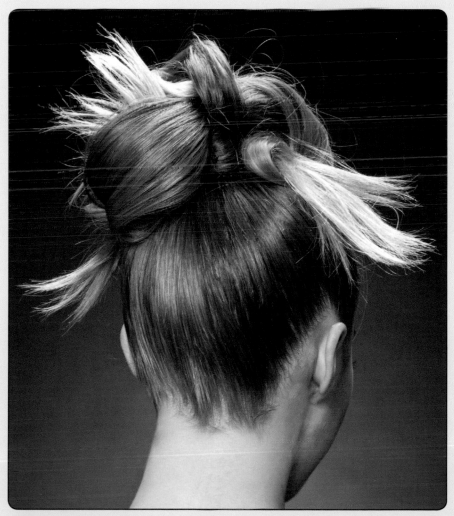

15

FUNKY FORMAL

UPDO

2

Straight hair is transformed into wavy and dramatic in this hairstyle, thanks to a carefully placed, long hair extension. Both the back and front of this design will draw double takes.

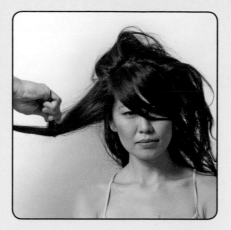

1

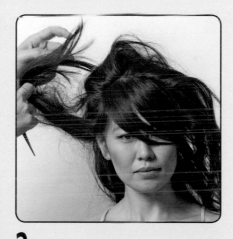

2

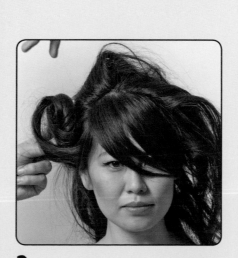

3

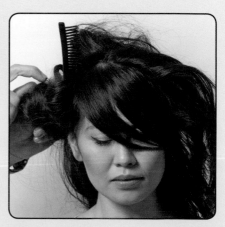

4

1. Wash and blow dry the hair. Grasp a section of hair above the ear on one side of the head and backcomb it.

2. Roll the hair upward with your fingers.

3. Roll the hair all the way to the roots, and secure it near the nape of the neck with bobby pins.

4. Make sure to keep the folded hair loose enough to maintain volume. Repeat this process with several sections of hair, moving in an arc over the crown of the head.

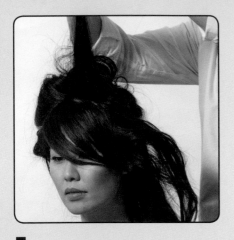

5.

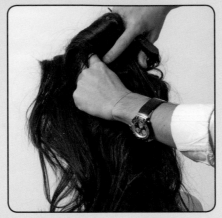

6.

5. Backcomb and roll each section of hair a bit differently, creating a look of asymmetrical volume in each roll.

6. Secure each roll near the base of the first roll at the back of the head.

7. Continue until you reach the other side of the head.

8. Remember to backcomb each section of hair, from the ends to the roots, for maximum volume.

9. Roll the hair gently using your fingers.

10. Rolling the hair loosely creates the desired casual look.

11. Secure the bangs, or leave them loose and swept across one side of the brow.

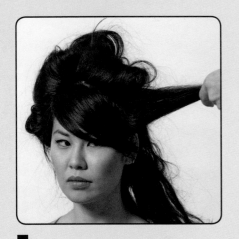

7.

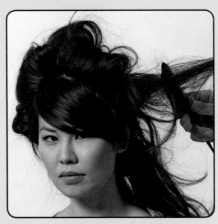

8.

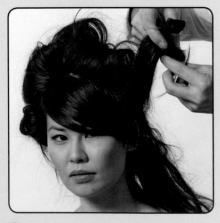

9.

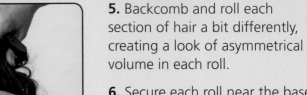

10.

11.

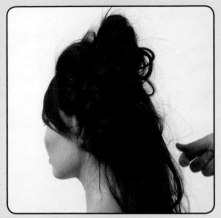

12

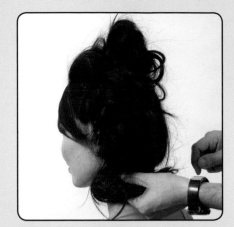

13

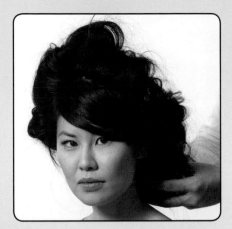

14

12. Roll the last lock of hair along the crown and secure it at the back of the head.

13. Backcomb the hair at the back of the neck, and roll it upward to leave an exposed neck.

14. Arrange the hair as desired, and mist it with holding spray.

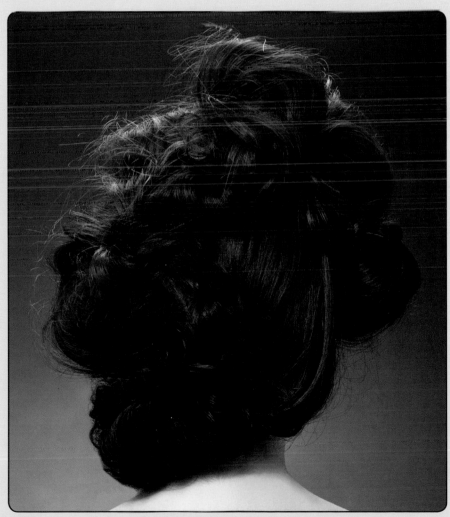

15

FREESTYLE

CRIMP

3

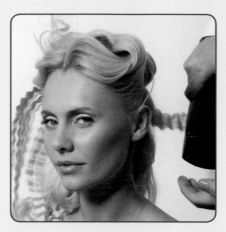

1

1. Wash the hair, apply styling mousse, and then blow dry. Gather ½-inch sections of hair and crimp them with a crimp iron, starting at the roots and working your way to the ends. For best results, hold the crimp iron for about 5 seconds each time.

2. Start with the hair at the back and bottom of the head, and work your way upward.

3. Crimp each lock, from the roots to the ends.

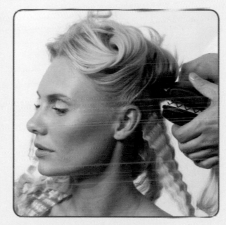

2

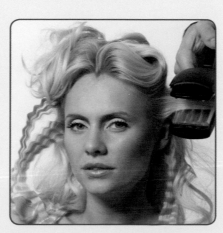

3

This carefree style can be as wild as you like. It is full of volume and velocity thanks to a crimp iron and lots of backcombing.

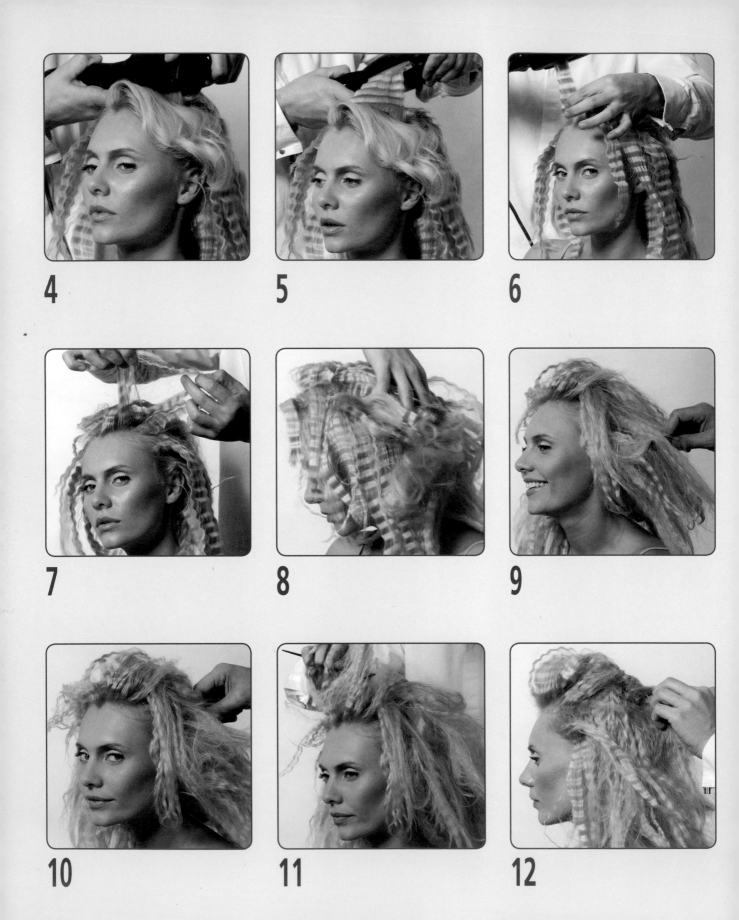

4

5

6

7

8

9

10

11

12

4. When all the hair at the bottom has been crimped, move your way to the top of the head and continue crimping the hair.

5. Crimp the hair from the root to the ends.

6. Continue this process for the remaining hair.

7. Run your fingers through the crimped sections of hair.

8. Run your fingers through the entire hairstyle to create wide and open crimped sections of hair.

9. Backcomb sections of hair at the root to create volume.

10. Repeat for all remaining hair.

11. Focus the backcombing on the roots so as not to damage the crimps.

12. Draw the bangs loosely to the back of the head, and secure them with bobby pins.

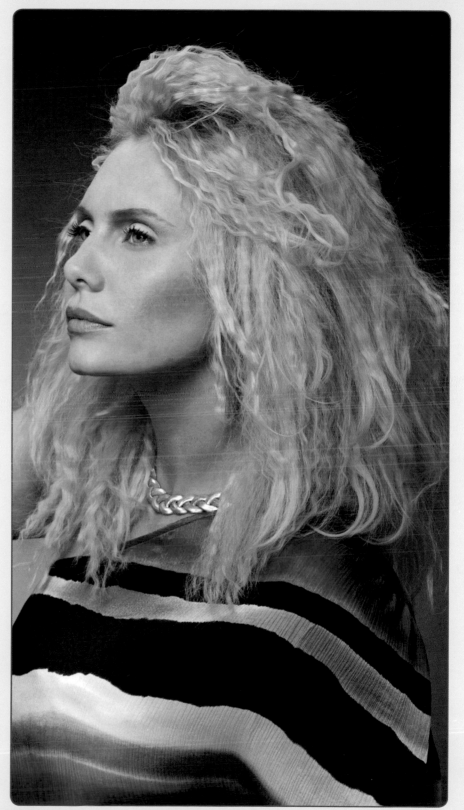

13

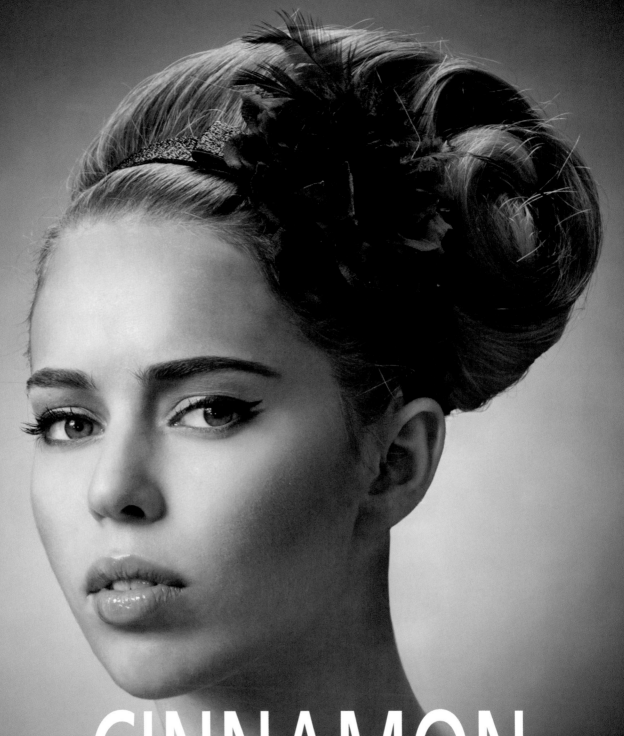

CINNAMON
SIDE TWIST

4

This high twist is located at the side of the head, creating an interestingly asymmetrical look. Add a daring hair band to complete the look.

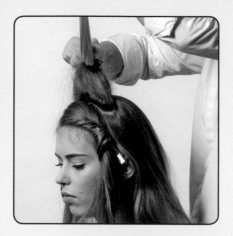

1

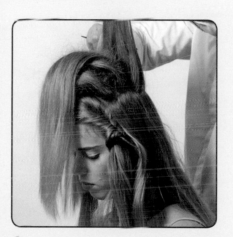

2

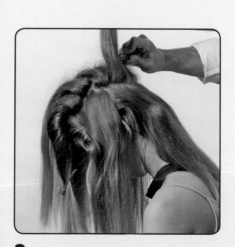

3

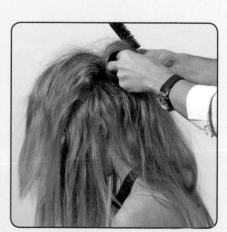

4

1. Wash and blow dry the hair. Make a part that extends from the front of each ear over the top of the crown. Backcomb the hair at the middle of the head, behind the part.

2. Continuing to backcomb 3-inch wide sections of hair at the middle of the head, from the top of the head toward the nape of the neck.

3. Mist each section of hair with holding spray after it is backcombed, before moving on to the next section.

4. Just below the crown, roll a section of hair around a large curler and secure with bobby pins.

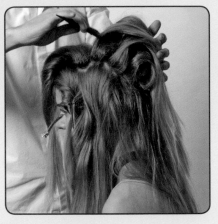

5

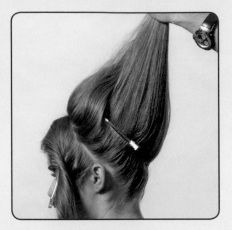

6

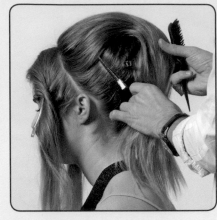

7

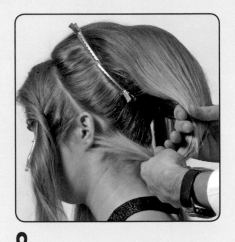

8

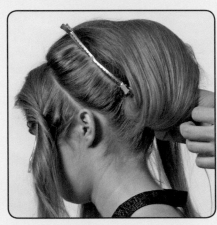

9

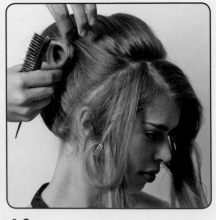

10

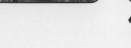

11

5. Gently comb back the hair in front of the curled section of hair, without losing volume.

6. Draw back the hair at the front and brush it together with the hair at the back of the head.

7. Secure the hair all around the bottom with bobby pins.

8. Brush the gathered hair and mist it with holding spray. Fold the hair downward at the back of the head, and secure the ends with an elastic band.

9. Affix the ends of the hair at the back of the head, so that the folded hair conceals the elastic band and the ends.

10. Draw out a lock from the gathered hair, twist it upward toward the center of the head, and secure it with a bobby pin.

11. Backcomb the hair at the front of the head.

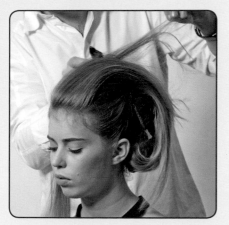

12

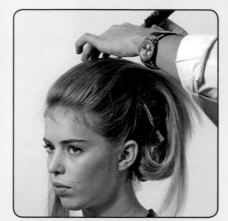

13

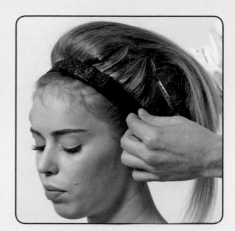

14

12. Brush the hair backward and combine it with the gathered hair. Mist the hair with holding spray as you comb it backward.

13. Secure the hair to the head with bobby pins.

14. Affix a band around the head, and attach a flower to one side.

15. Tuck in the loose ends and secure them with bobby pins.

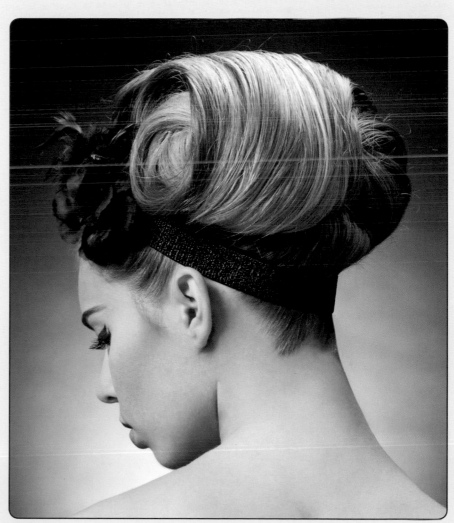

15

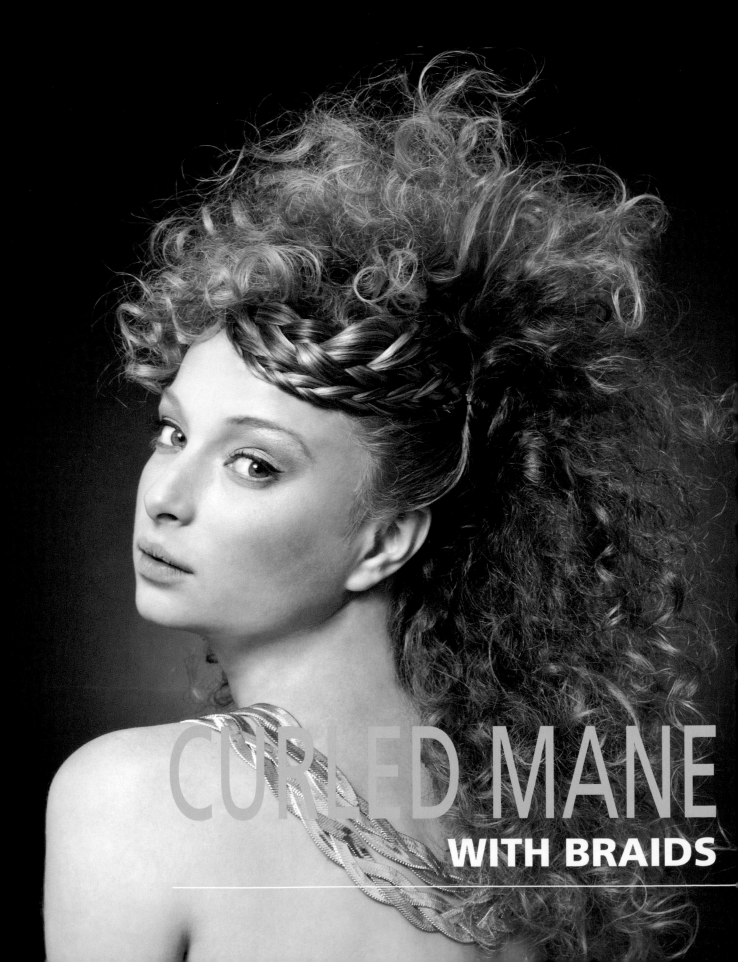

CURLED MANE
WITH BRAIDS

5

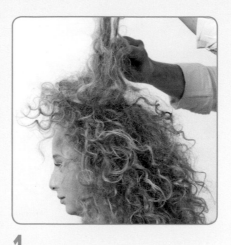

1

1. Wash and blow dry the hair curly. Backcomb the hair at the crown.

2. Continue to backcomb all the hair to increase volume.

3. Comb back the hair at one side of the head, from behind the ear to the front of the head, toward the crown.

4. Comb only the roots of the hair, leaving the curls untouched.

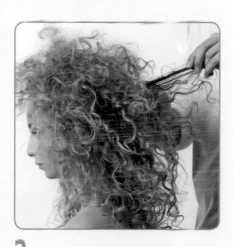

2

The braided tiara at the front of this hairstyle is a spectacular contrast with the intense curls at the back. The combination is breathtaking.

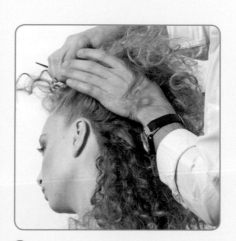

3

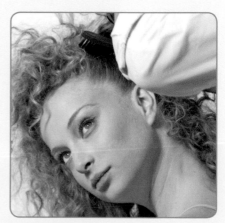

4

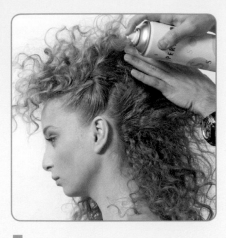

5

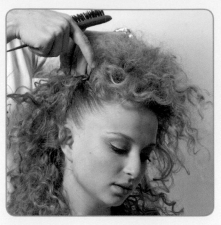

6

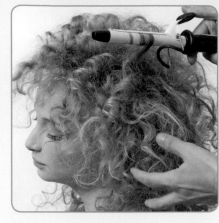

7

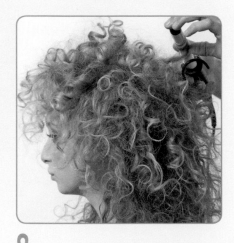

8

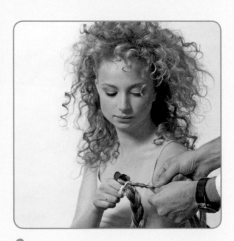

9

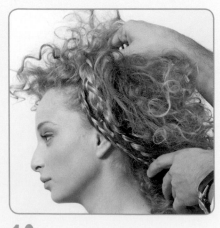

10

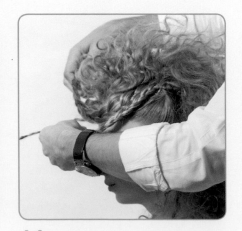

11

5. Twist the combed hair gently; then secure it with bobby pins. Mist with holding spray to secure.

6. Repeat this process on the opposite side.

7. Using a curling iron, restore any curls that were damaged by the combing.

8. Use the curling iron to make curls that are softer and rounder than your natural hair texture.

9. Select a long hair extension that matches the color of the hair, and fold it in half. Divide both halves into three sections each and make two braids. Secure the braids with an elastic band at the end.

10. Attach the braided extension above one ear, over the gathered hair, with bobby pins.

11. Draw the braids across the front of the head, toward the other ear.

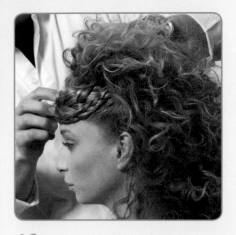

12

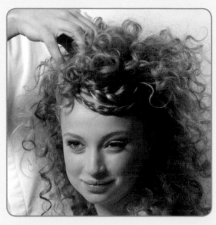

13

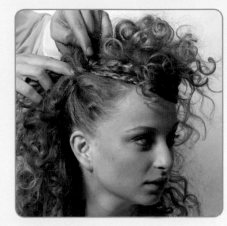

14

12. Secure the other end of the braids at the other side of the head, over the gathered hair.

13. Arrange the braids over the brow, so that they hang gently and contrast nicely with the wild, curled hair at the back.

14. Adjust the bobby pins where the braids are secured, so that the same pins hold the braids and the gathered hair.

15. Backcomb all curls to maximize volume and create a wild look. Mist with holding spray to secure.

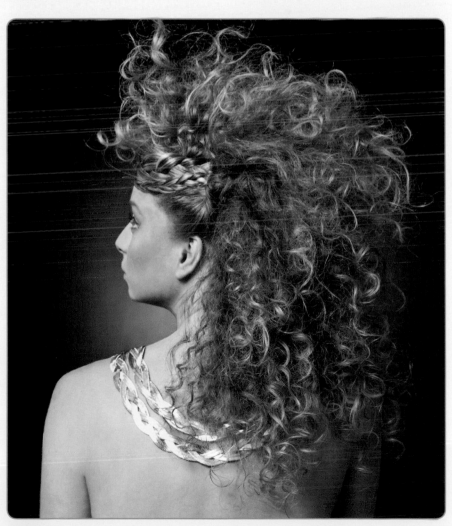

15

CURLS
OF COLOR

6

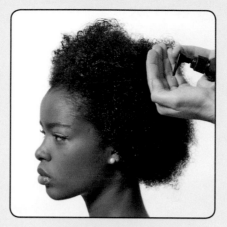

1

1. Wash the hair and towel dry. Apply styling gel to the hair.

2. After the styling gel is distributed evenly, apply moisturizing cream to the hair.

3. Place a bit of moisturizing cream in your hands and scrunch the hair to disperse the cream evenly, all the way to the roots.

4. Comb together a few locks of hair.

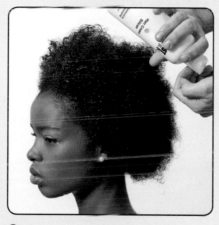

2

This hairstyle is full of pizzazz. Use any color hair extension you like, or try a combination of colors for a really striking effect.

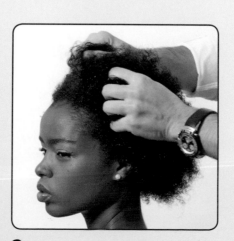

3

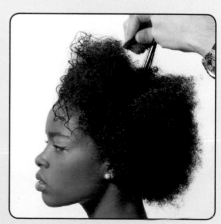

4

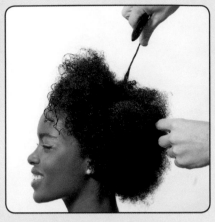

5

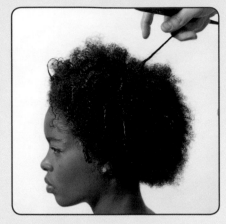

6

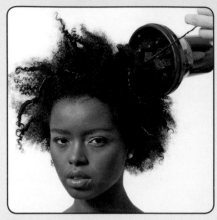

7

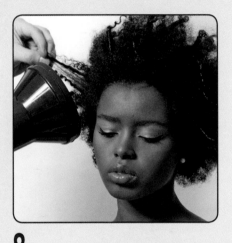

8

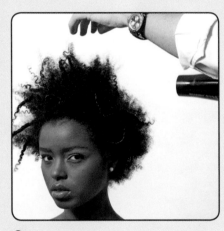

9

5. Twist the locks together to form a tight curl.

6. Repeat this process for all remaining hair, separating the locks before twisting them into a curl.

7. Blow dry the hair with a diffuser.

8. Tug gently at the curls as you dry them to open them up a bit and add length.

9. After the curls have been lengthened, blow dry the hair without the diffuser.

10. Attach a colorful hair extension to a hairpin and twist it into a curl. Blow dry the extension, and mist it with holding spray.

11. When the curl is secured, release the extension from the hair pin.

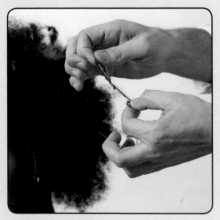

10

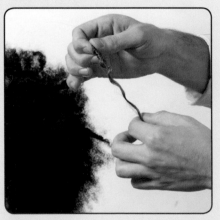

11

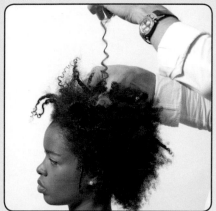

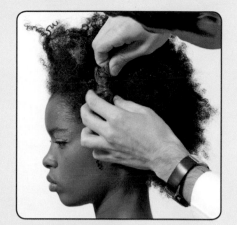

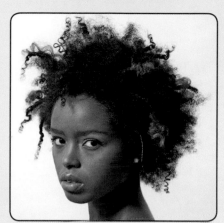

12

13

14

12. Measure a length of extension alongside a length of hair, and cut the extension to the desired length.

13. Attach the extension to a bobby pin and secure it close to the roots.

14. Repeat this process with as many hair extensions as you like, spacing the extensions evenly around the head. Use extensions of the same color or different colors.

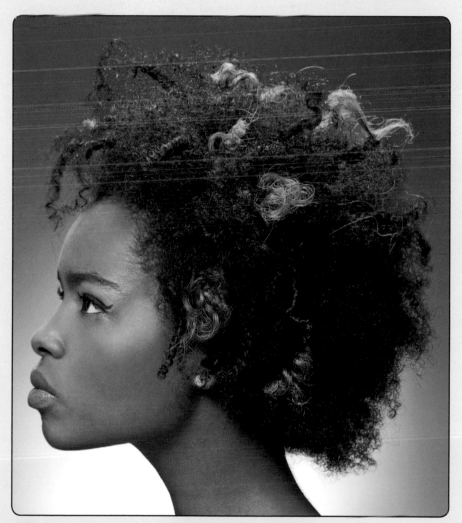

15

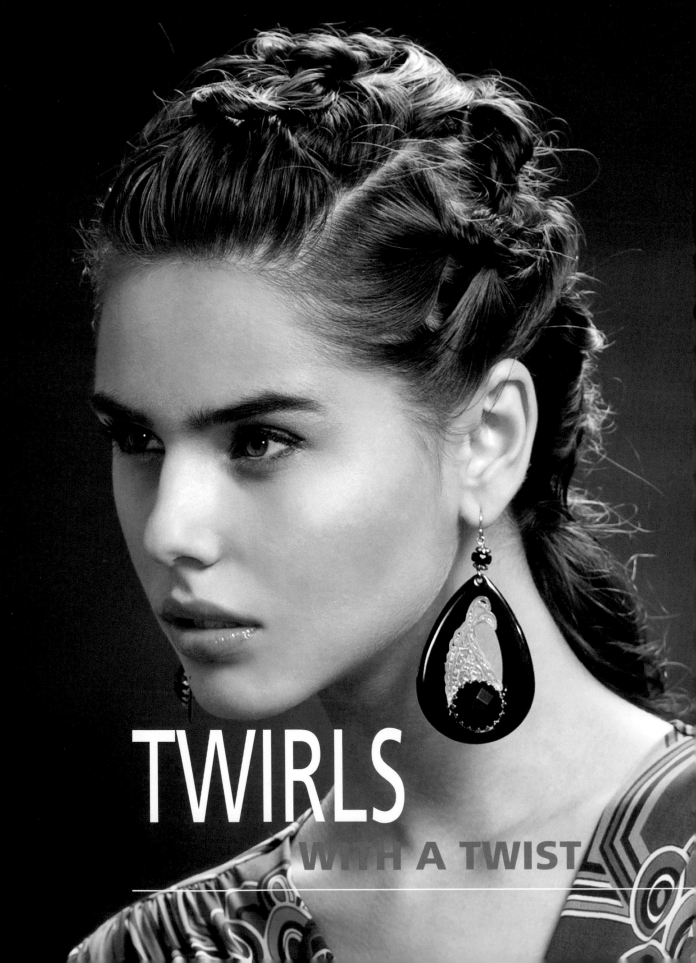

TWIRLS

WITH A TWIST

7

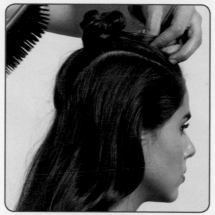

1

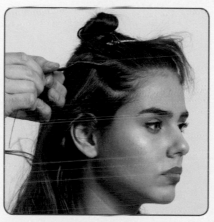

2

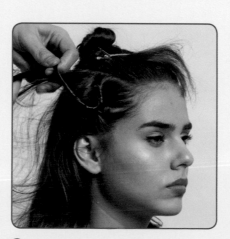

3

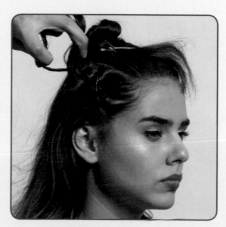

4

1. Wash and blow dry the hair. Make two parts that extend from the brow to the crown to separate the hair into three even sections. Gather the hair in the middle section in a bun at the crown of the head.

2. Gather a 1-inch wide lock of hair to the right of the right side part, and twist it into a tight rope.

3. Gather a second 1-inch lock of hair from behind the first lock and twist them together.

4. Continue to gather 1-inch locks of hair, each time connecting the new one with the previous one.

The front of this hairstyle features several twisted locks. At the back, the hair is twisted together in a thick, sweeping whirlwind of a finish.

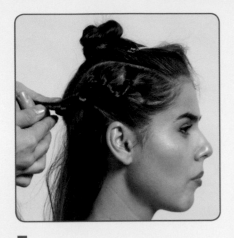

5

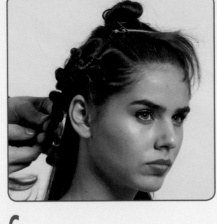

6

5. Repeat to create a single twisted rope of hair at one side of the head.

6. When you reach the ear line, secure the twisted lock temporarily with a clip.

7. Move to the middle section of hair and repeat the process, starting with a 1-inch wide lock of hair at the brow.

8. Be sure to pull the hair back as you twist it, to maintain a tight twisted form. At this stage, the twisted hair should resemble a snake.

9. When you reach an area that is parallel to the ear line, join the middle section of hair with the rightmost section of hair by twisting the two sections together.

10. Move to the leftmost section of hair and repeat the process. Gather all three sections of hair at the back of the head, below the crown.

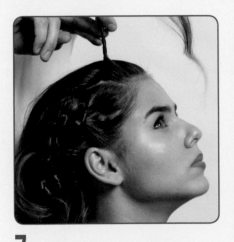

7

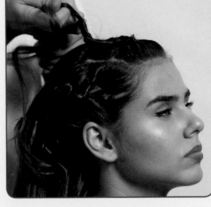

8

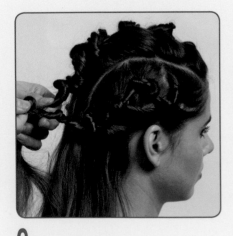

9

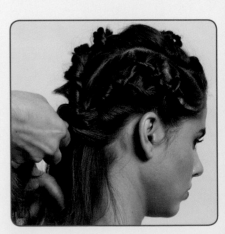

10

11

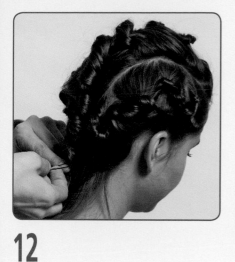

12

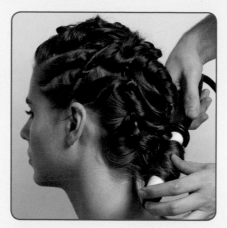

13

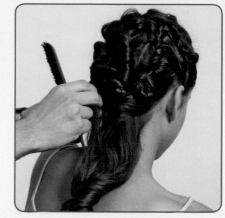

14

11. Braid the loose hair at the back of the head by collecting locks from each side of the head and integrating them into a braid in the middle.

12. Continue braiding until you reach the nape of the neck; then secure the hair at the nape of the neck with a pin.

13. Roll all the loose hair into a curl with a medium curling iron.

14. To complete the look, separate a lock of hair from the large curl at the back, wrap it around the hair at the base of the neck, and secure with bobby pins. Mist with holding spray to secure.

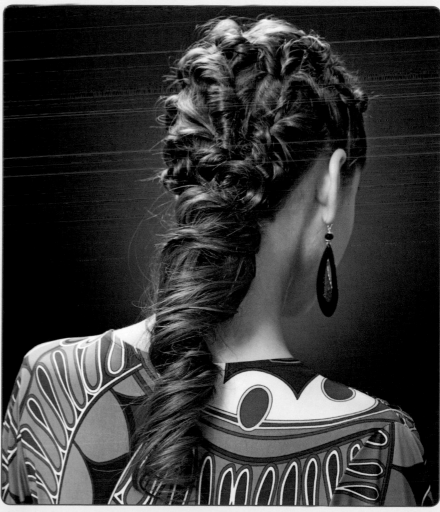

15

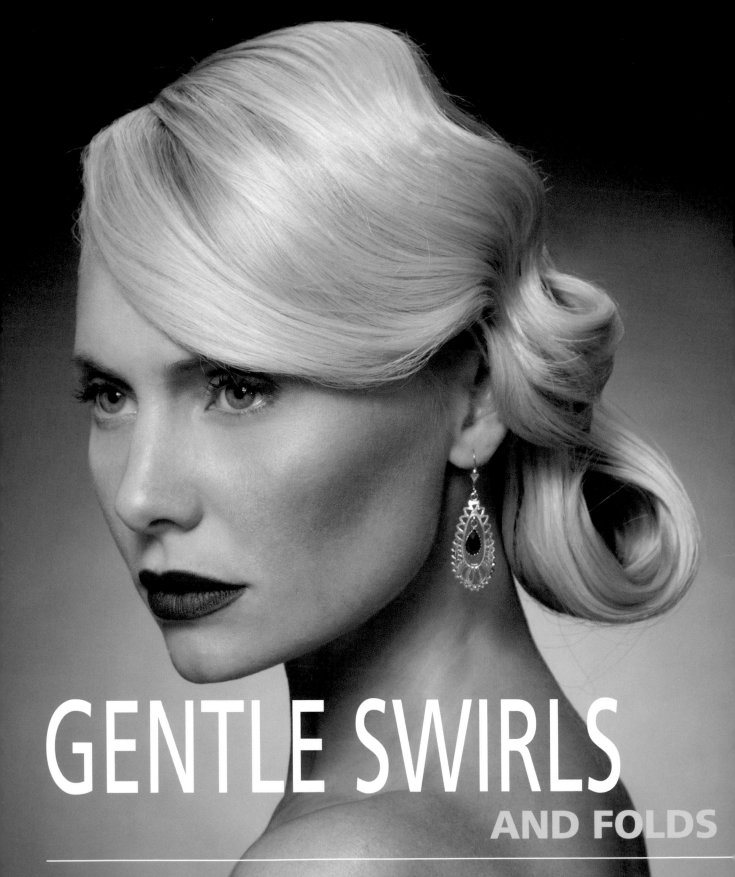

GENTLE SWIRLS
AND FOLDS

8

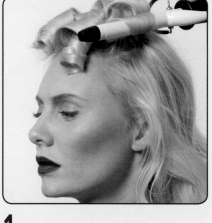

1

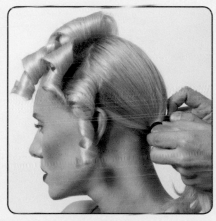

2

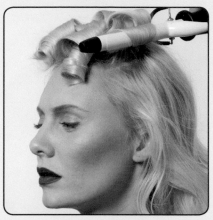

3

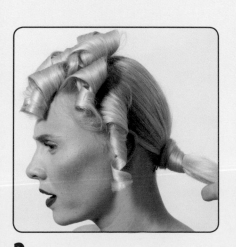

4

1. Wash and blow dry the hair. Make a part from the top of each ear over the crown, and curl the hair above this part, section by section, with a small curling iron.

2. Gather the loose hair in a low ponytail at the nape of the neck, and secure it with an elastic band.

3. Wrap a lock of hair from the ponytail around the elastic band to conceal it, and secure it with bobby pins.

4. Comb out the curls at the front of the head.

The bangs in this hairstyle are gently draped over one eye to create an asymmetrical front. At the back, the hair is collected into a softly folded ponytail behind one ear.

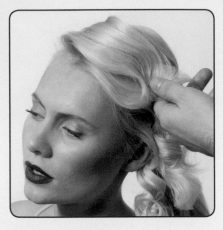

5

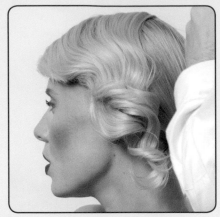

6

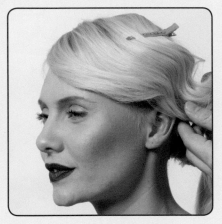

7

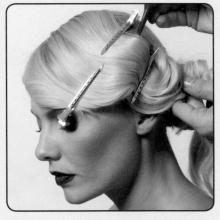

8

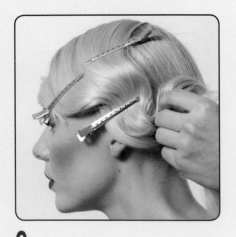

9

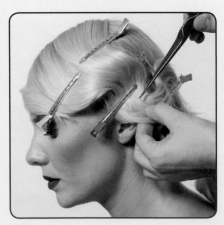

10

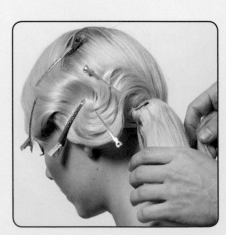

11

5. Make a deep side part at the front of the head, and comb the curls to one side.

6. Brush the curled hair together and draw it backward along one side.

7. Affix the hair along the side of the head with bobby pins. Allow the hair to flow with the wavy lines created by the curls.

8. For extra volume, pull the hair away from the head in the areas between the clips.

9. Once your hair is in the desired position, add clips to secure it.

10. Mist the hair with holding spray, and wait for 10 minutes for it to set.

11. Select a hair extension that matches the color of the hair, and affix it at the base of the ponytail to add length and volume.

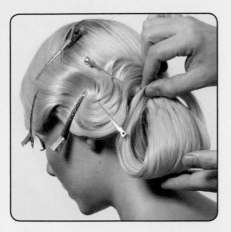

12

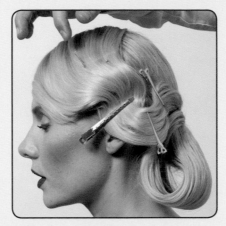

13

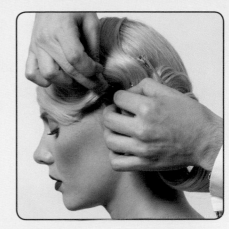

14

12. Fold the ponytail inward, toward the nape of the neck, and secure the ends at each side of the ponytail base with bobby pins.

13. Make sure the holding spray is dry and the waves secure before replacing the clips with bobby pins.

14. Work gradually to replace all the clips with bobby pins. Make sure the waves are secure before removing the clips.

15. Mist the hair with holding spray to finish.

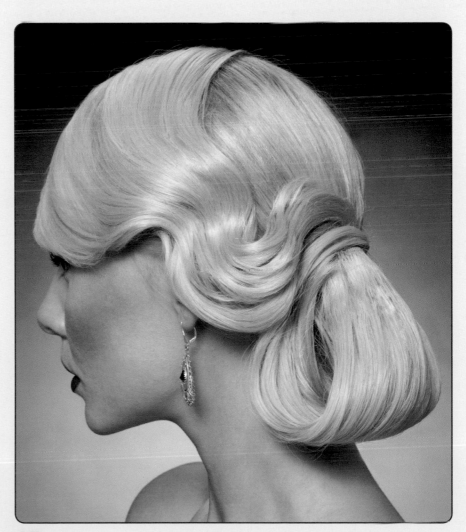

15

STRIKING
SPIKES

9

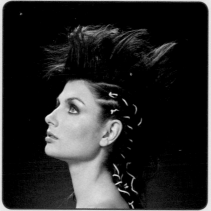

1

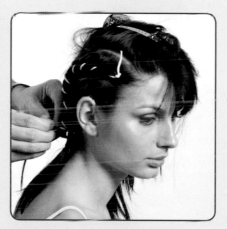

2

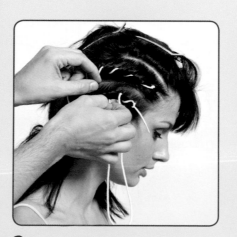

3

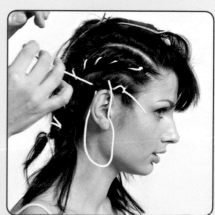

4

1. Wash and blow dry the hair. Attach a colorful hair extension to a lock of hair at the roots.

2. Make several parts that extend from the brow to the neck. Twist the hair in each section into a rope, and secure at the nape of the neck with a clip. Tie a string around the rope of hair near the front of the section, and wrap the string around the rope. Tie the string near the nape of the neck.

3. Repeat the process with another section of hair.

4. Wrap the string around the rope of hair.

If you like to stand out, then this hairstyle is just right for you. It combines several techniques and accessories for a look that is unique and striking.

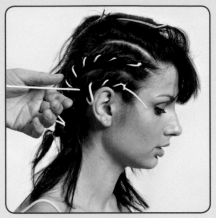

5

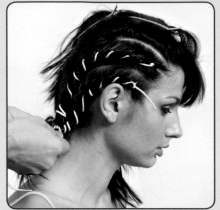

6

5. Continue wrapping the string around the hair until you reach the nape of the neck.

6. Tie the string in a knot at the nape of the neck, and cut off the excess string.

7. Repeat this process on the other side of the head, leaving the hair on the top of the head loose. Mist the loose hair with holding spray.

8. Backcomb the loose hair near the brow.

9. Mist the loose hair with holding spray while backcombing it upward, to create a messy look.

10. For a strong hold, make sure the hair in the middle is backcombed all the way to the roots.

11. Continue this process all the way to the nape of the neck.

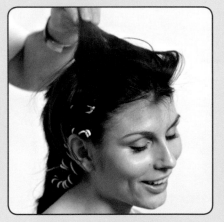

7

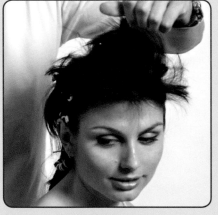

8

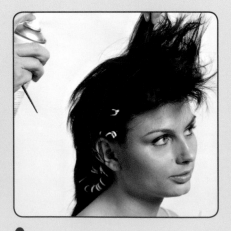

9

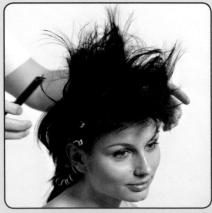

10

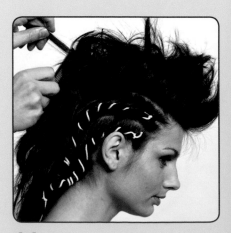

11

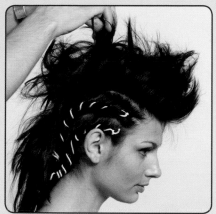

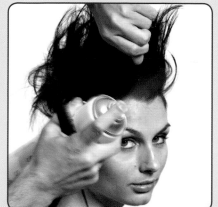

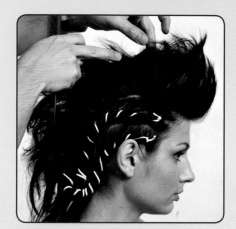

12

13

14

12. Adjust the hair along the middle of head to add height.

13. To ensure a strong hold, mist the hair with holding spray

14. Secure sections of hair in the middle to the head with bobby pins.

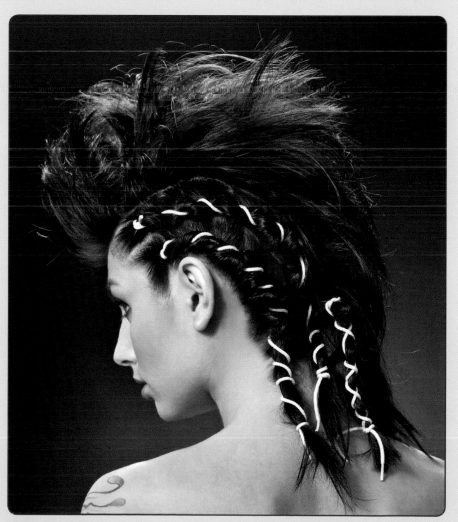

15

LONG
AND LUSCIOUS

10

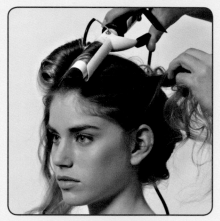

1

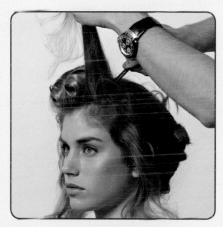

2

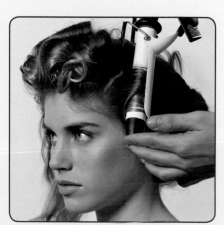

3

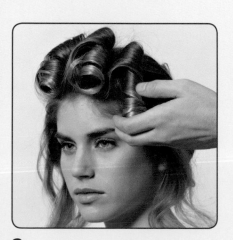

4

1. Wash and blow dry the hair straight. Divide the hair from the brow to the crown into sections, and curl each section with a medium curling iron.

2. Backcomb each section of hair before curling it, for maximum volume.

3. Continue to make curls all along the brow line.

4. Make the curls as close to the root as possible.

This enticing hairstyle is high on volume and style. Make it as long as you like according to the hair extension you select.

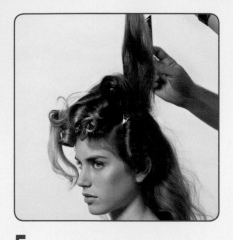

5

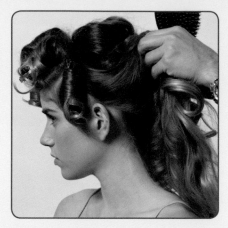

6

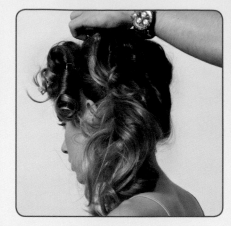

7

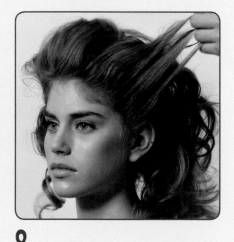

8

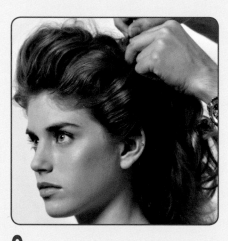

9

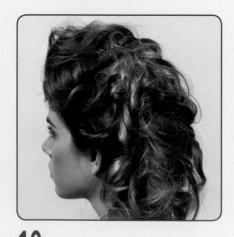

10

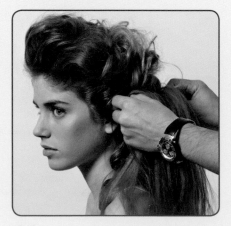

11

5. Backcomb the hair below the crown upward and over the crown.

6. Loosely gather the hair at the sides of the head toward the backcombed base.

7. Draw the hair backward and toward one side of the head, and secure it with clips.

8. Gently release the curls at the front of the head, combing them gently with your fingers.

9. Draw the hair at the brow upward and backward to maintain volume and height at the front of the head. Secure with bobby pins at the crown of the head.

10. Be sure to secure the hair in a manner that looks natural and tousled.

11. Select a hair extension that matches the natural color of the hair. Attach the extension under the hair at the back of the head to create extra length and volume.

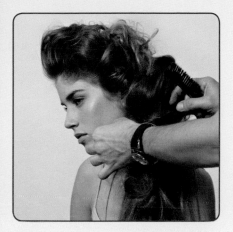

12

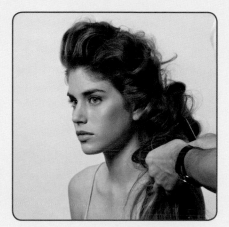

13

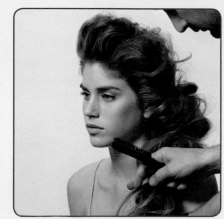

14

12. Backcomb the extension for a dramatic effect.

13. Grasp small sections of hair in the hair extension and backcomb the hair to increase volume. You may want to use tiny elastic bands to secure the small sections of hair.

14. Arrange the hair so that it has a wild, windblown look. Bring the hair over one shoulder, and mist it with holding spray to secure.

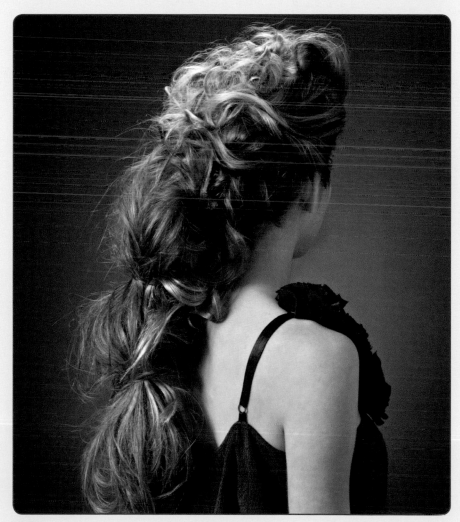

15

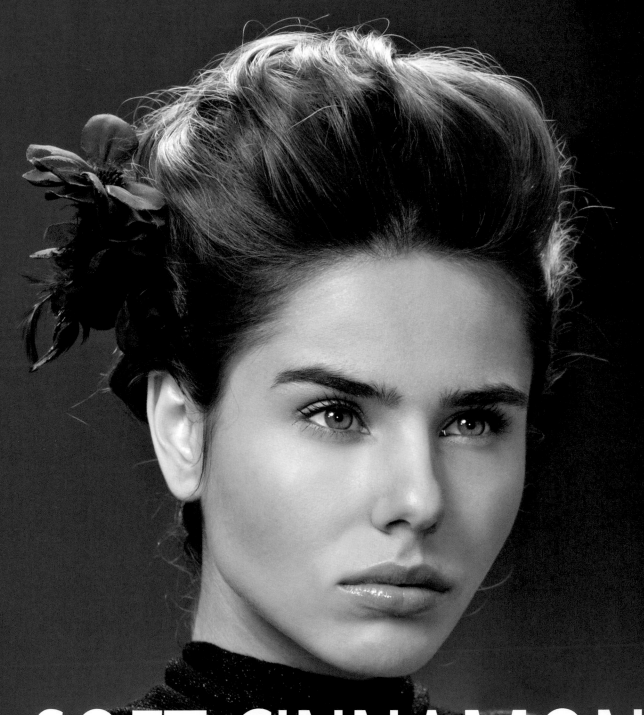

SOFT CINNAMON
BUN

11

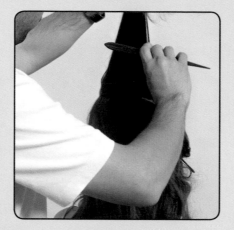

1

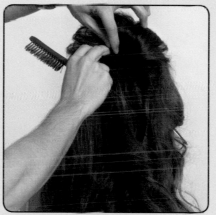

2

Lift your hair (and spirits) with this soft curly updo. It has a gentle and high front, and a dramatic but soft back. This hairstyle is excellent for day or night.

1. Wash and blow dry the hair. Curl the hair with a large curling iron. Gather a 3-inch long section of hair along the brow and backcomb it to create volume.

2. Draw the backcombed hair backward and secure at the crown with a hairpin. This hair serves as the base for shaping the rest of the hair.

3. Gather the hair on one side of the head and twist it toward the crown in a coil. Secure it with bobby pins. To maintain volume, avoid pulling the hair too tightly.

4. Gather the hair on the other side of the head and twist it toward the crown. Secure it with bobby pins.

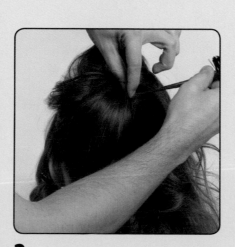

3

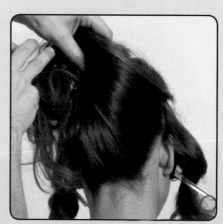

4

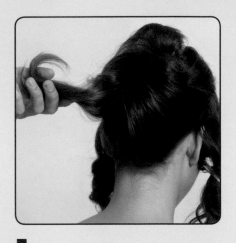

5

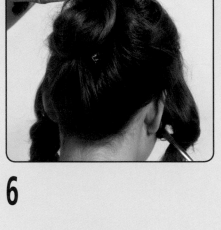

6

5. Mist the loose ends with holding spray.

6. Twist together the loose ends and roll the lock toward the coil at the crown. Secure it with bobby pins.

7. The coil is created from thick, loosely fastened locks of hair.

8. Gently comb the backcombed hair at the top to create a wave.

9. Gently lift the roots of the secured backcombed hair to maintain the volume, and secure the hair close to the root to create height.

10. Comb back the bangs and hold the ends tightly at an upward angle. Position the holding spray about 6 inches away and mist the ends.

11. Loosen your grip on the ends and allow the hair to return to a loose, natural wave.

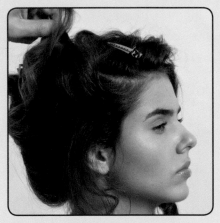

7

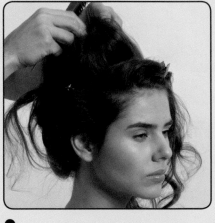

8

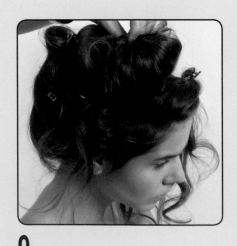

9

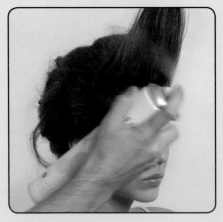

10

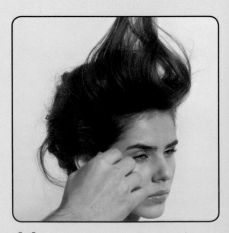

11

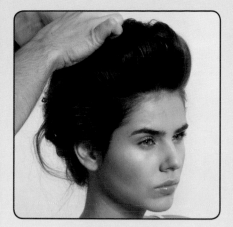

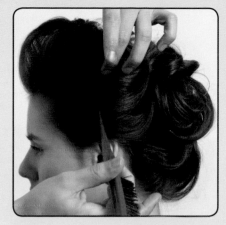

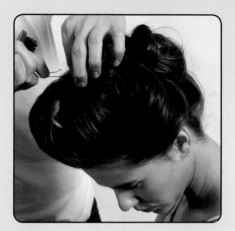

12

13

14

12. Secure the end of the lock to the crown with a bobby pin.

13. Go through the hair and separate tightened locks with the tip of a comb for a gentle, unified finish. Mist the hair with holding spray.

14. For a polished finish, lift the secured bangs a bit higher and secure them with bobby pins.

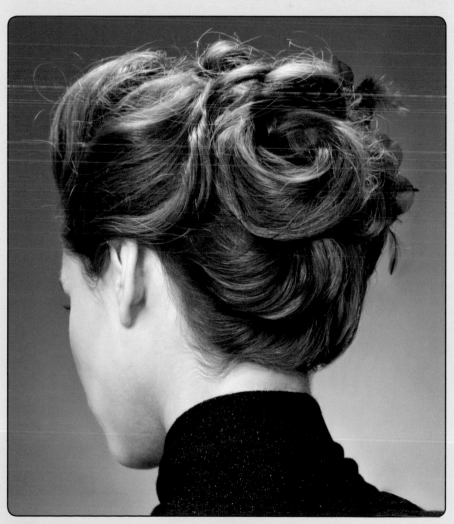

15

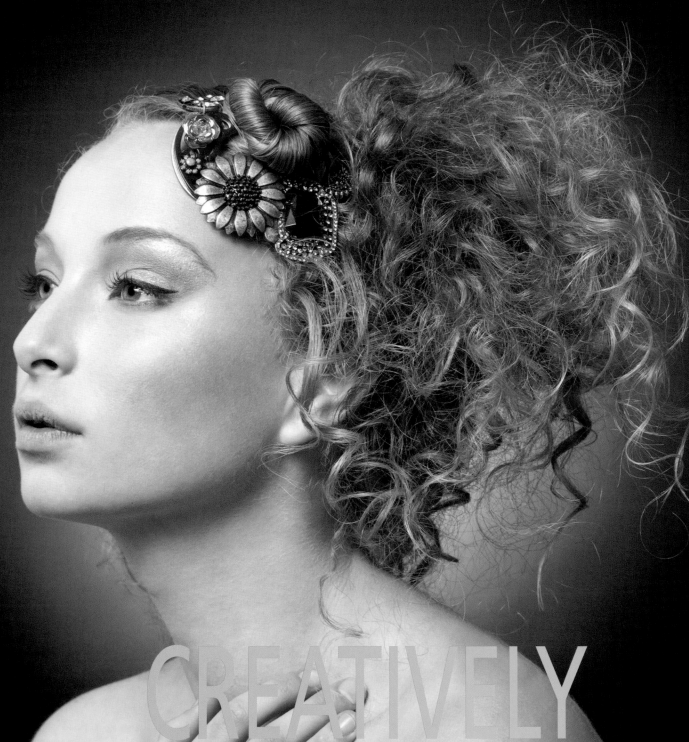

CREATIVELY

CURLY

12

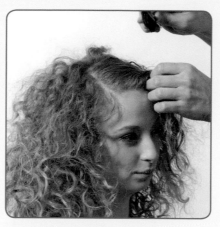

1

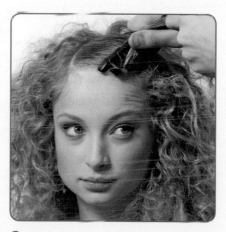

2

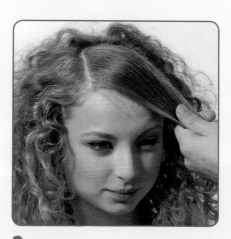

3

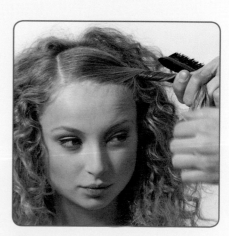

4

1. Wash and towel dry the hair. Apply moisturizing cream with your hands, and dry hair with a diffuser.

2. Gather a square section of hair from the front of the brow to the top of the crown.

3. Wet the hair in this section, and then comb it forward to straighten it.

4. Draw the hair to the side and twist it tightly around itself.

This playful look features asymmetrical, curly ponytails. The addition of a stone-studded hair accessory adds a polished element to this otherwise wild design.

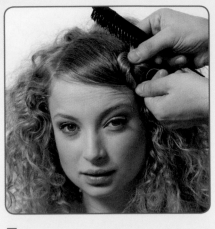

5

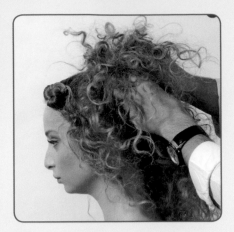

6

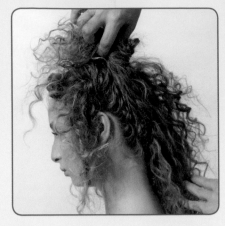

7

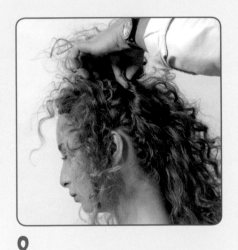

8

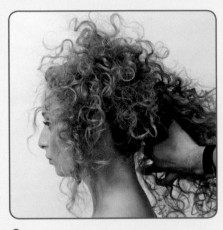

9

5. Wrap the twisted hair into a bun, and tie it in a knot at the end to keep it in place.

6. Shape the back of the hair with your hands, adjusting the height as desired.

7. Divide the hair at the back into a top and bottom section. Collect the hair at the top and twist it upward.

8. Secure the twisted hair with a clip, leaving the ends loose and dangling forward at one side.

9. Lift the bottom section of hair at the back of the head in the opposite direction, twisting it upward.

10. Secure this section of hair, leaving the ends loose and dangling forward to create a playful, asymmetrical look.

11. Enhance some of the curls at the back by tightening them with a small curling iron.

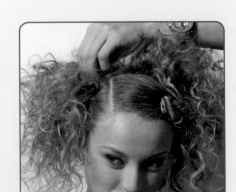

10

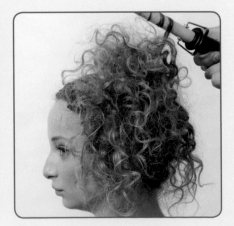

11

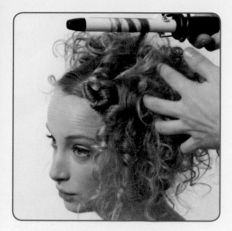

12

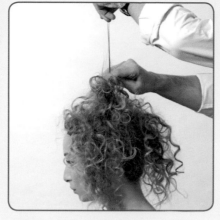

13

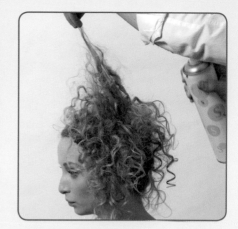

14

12. Curl some of the locks at the front as well, to provide a contrast with the straight hair at the front.

13. For extra volume, grasp the ends of some locks with one hand and backcomb the hair with your other hand, toward the roots.

14. Mist the hair with holding spray to secure the curls in a lively and carefree arrangement.

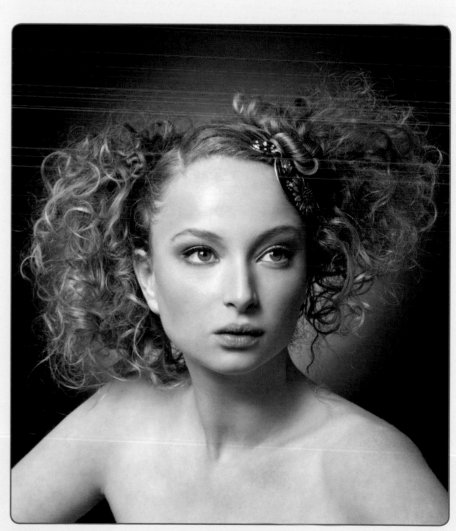

15

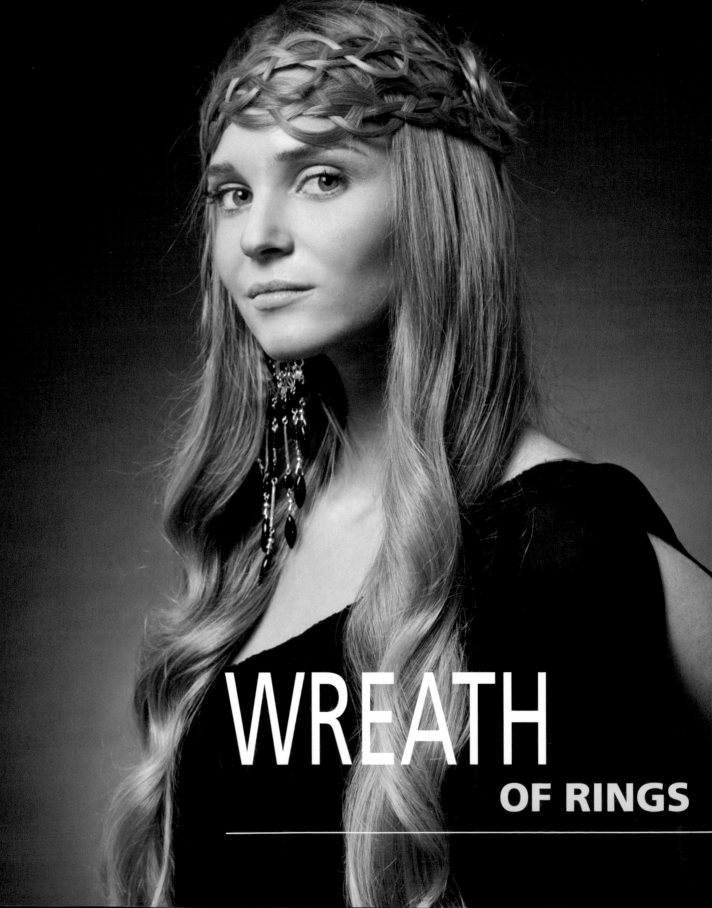

WREATH
OF RINGS

13

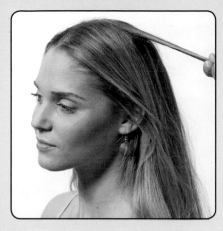

1

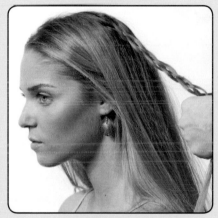

2

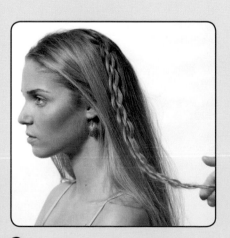

3

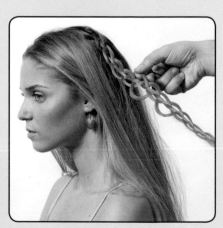

4

This delicate hairstyle features elaborate-looking braided rings made with natural, long hair. The rings encircling the head contrast beautifully with the long, loose locks.

1. Wash and blow dry the hair straight. Make a middle part from the front of the hair to the crown, and select a lock of hair beside the part, at the crown.

2. Divide the lock into four sections and braid them together loosely to make a four-strand braid. To do this, number each section of hair from 1 to 4. Pass strand 2 over strand 1, and strand 3 over strand 4. Pass the new strand 2 over strand 3 to make an X in the middle of the strands. Now pass the new strand 2 over strand 1, and the new strand 3 over strand 4. Pass the new strand 2 over strand 3 to make an X in the middle of the strands.

3. Continue in this manner, braiding the hair until you reach the ends.

4. Hold the end of the braid, and gently tug on the loops to widen the braid. Secure the braid with an elastic band.

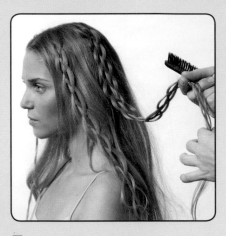

5

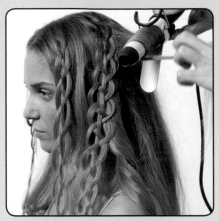

6

5. Select a lock of hair beside the part near the front of the head, divide it into four sections, and braid. Repeat the process with two locks of hair on the other side of the part.

6. Curl the loose hair into curls with a medium curling iron. Hold each lock in the curling iron for about 10 seconds.

7. Repeat this process to curl all the loose hair.

8. Grasp one of the braids at the crown of the head, and arrange the loops so that its structure is accentuated.

9. Draw the braid around to the front of the head, and wrap it across the brow.

10. With bobby pins, secure the end of the braid to the base of the front braid on the other side of the head.

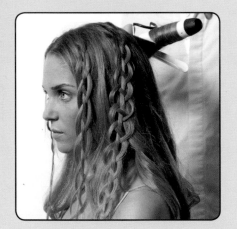

7

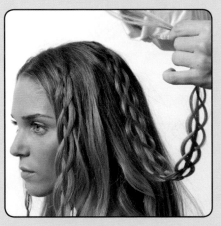

8

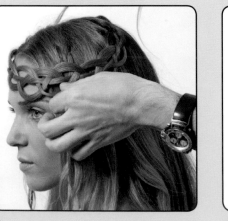

9

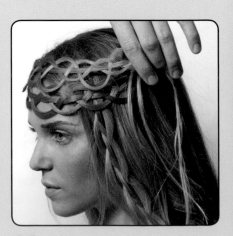

10

11

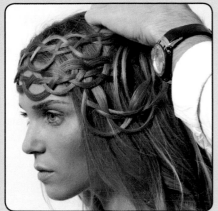

12

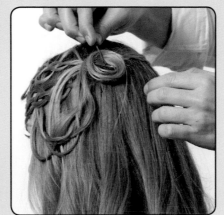

13

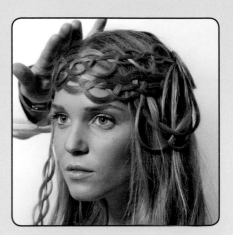

14

11. Repeat this process with the other braid that starts at the crown of the head, wrapping it in the opposite direction and securing it at the base of the back braid on the other side of the head.

12. Fold the front braid on this side of the head into a loop, and draw it toward the back braid on the same side of the head.

13. Roll the ends of hair into a loop, and secure the loop with bobby pins.

14. Let the front braid on the other side of the head hang down freely. Comb the loose hair for a soft and flowing finish.

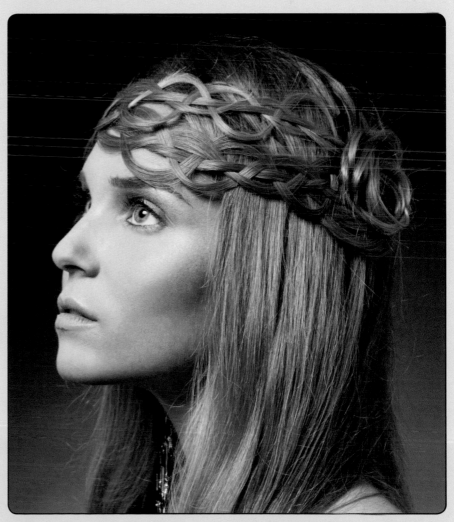

15

BRAIDED
CROWN

14

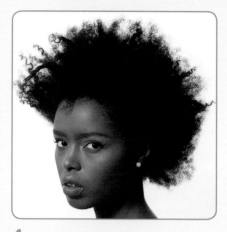

1

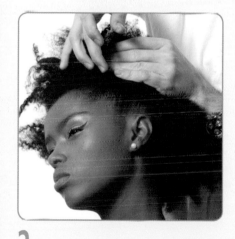

2

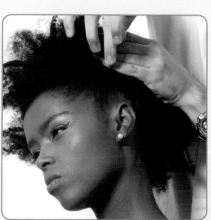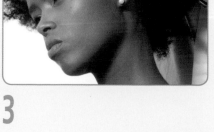

3

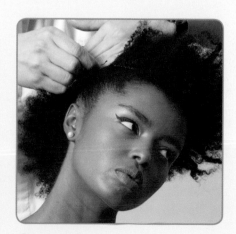

4

1. Wash the hair and towel dry. Apply moisturizing cream; then dry with a diffuser.

2. Brush all the hair on one side of the head upward, toward the crown.

3. Secure the hair upward with bobby pins and mist with holding spray.

4. Repeat this process on the opposite side.

You'll look (and feel) like royalty with this hairstyle. Natural hair is used for the upper area of the crown, while a long braided hair extension encircles the hairline.

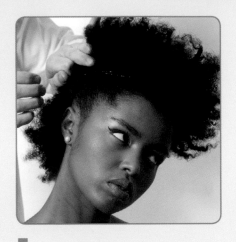

5

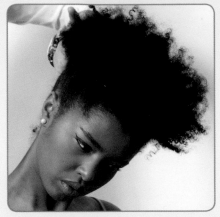

6

5. Comb the hair at the roots only to avoid damaging the natural curls.

6. Brush the hair at the back of the head upward, toward the crown.

7. Select a long hair extension that matches the color of the hair, and divide the extension into three sections. Braid the sections and secure at the end with an elastic band.

8. Attach the hair extension at one side of the head.

9. Draw the braid across the forehead and toward the other side of the head.

10. Draw the braid along the hairline, or just above it.

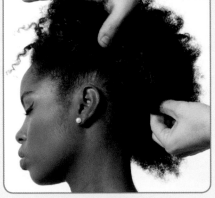

7

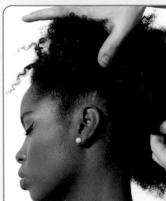

8

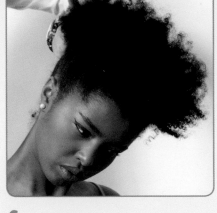

9

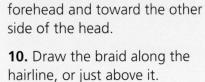

10

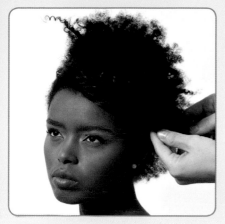

11

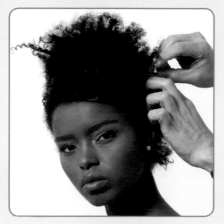

12

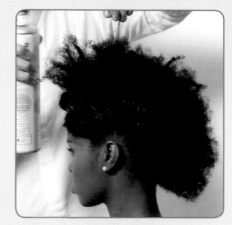

13

11. Secure the braid on the other side of the head with bobby pins.

12. For extra strength, secure the braid near the bobby pins that are holding up the natural hair.

13. Mist the hair with holding spray, and use your fingers to shape the curls at the top of the head.

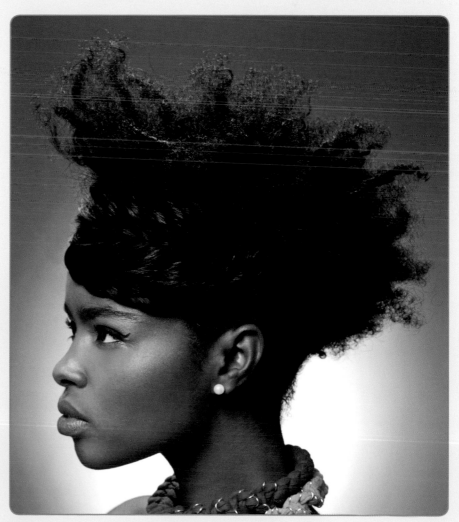

14

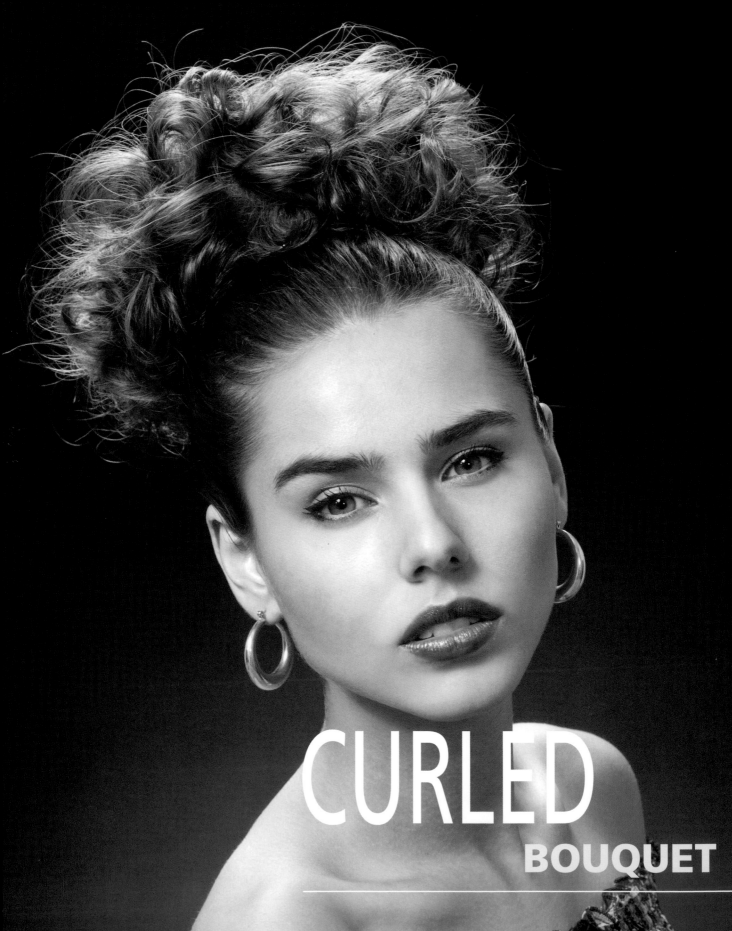

CURLED

BOUQUET

15

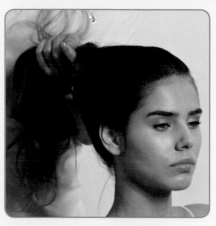

1

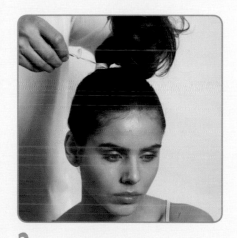

2

This hairstyle features a sleek and smooth front paired with a curled, wild back. Dramatic yet elegant, it combines a captivatingly curled bun with an alluringly bare neck.

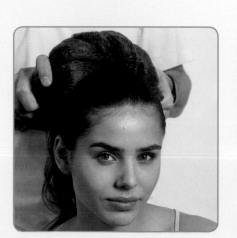

3

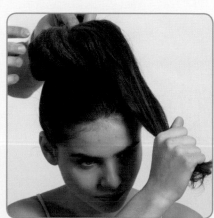

4

1. Wash and blow dry the hair with an inward wave toward the ends.

2. Gather the hair in a high ponytail.

3. Select a sponge that matches the color of the hair and shape it into a long and narrow sausage that can be wrapped around the entire base of the ponytail.

4. Wrap the sponge around the base of the ponytail.

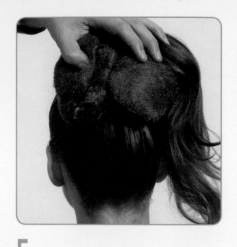

5

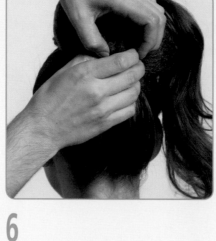

6

5. Make sure the ends of the sponge meet at the back of the head, under the ponytail.

6. Attach the sponge securely with bobby pins.

7. Draw a lock of hair from the ponytail and twist it around itself.

8. Hold the twisted lock at the tip and tug gently at the ends.

9. Slowly draw the hair in toward the head while releasing it from your grip, to form a coil.

10. Let the coil contract to form a curl while still holding a few strands of hair.

11. Draw the curled hair over the sponge to cover it, and secure the hair with a pin.

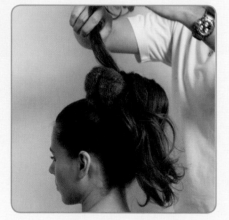

7

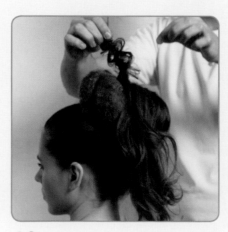

8

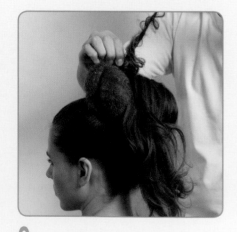

9

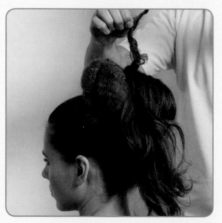

10

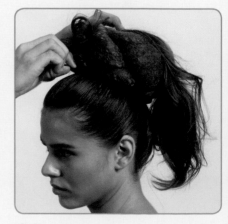

11

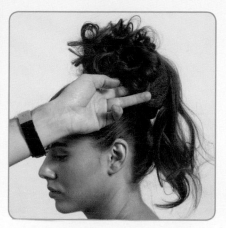

12

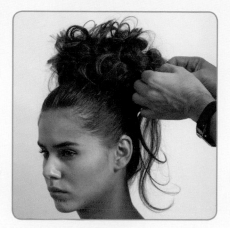

13

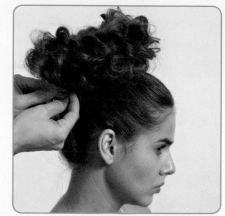

14

12. Repeat this technique with the remaining hair, separating the ponytail into strands, shaping each strand into a coil, and securing the coils all around the sponge. When pinning the hair into place, make sure that the locks conceal the sponge completely.

13. For extra strength, secure some locks of hair to the sponge as well.

14. Affix hair all around the sponge. Position the holding spray about 6 inches away and mist the hair.

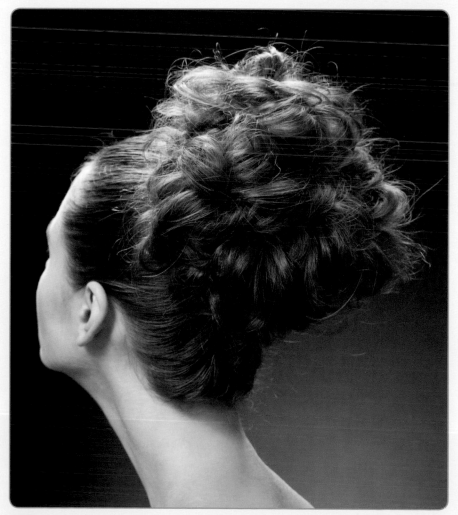

15

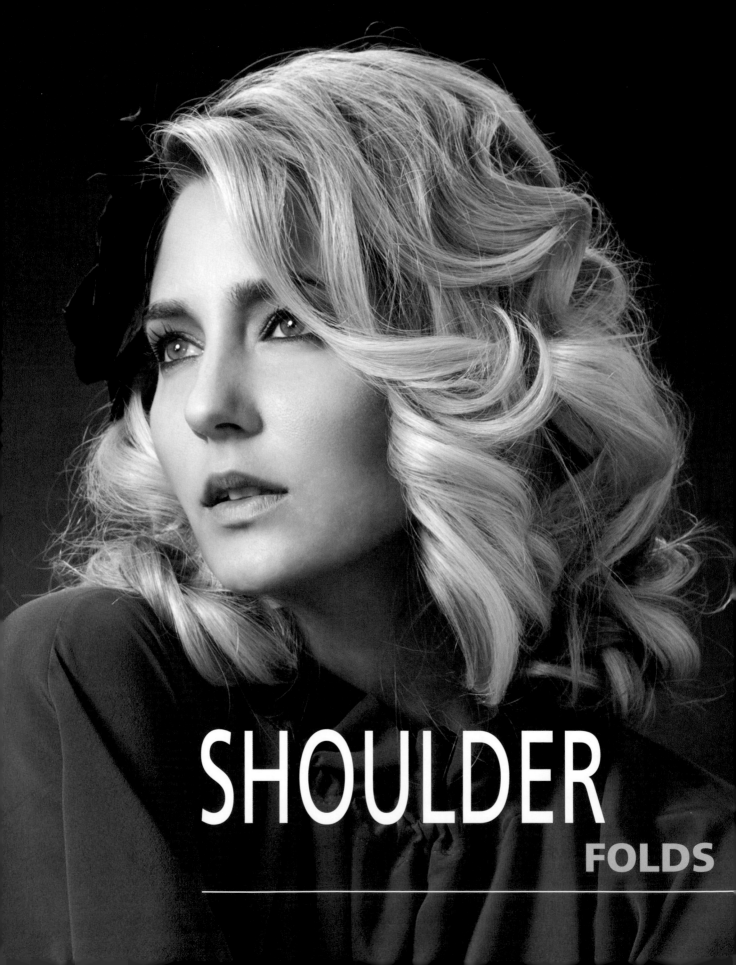

SHOULDER
FOLDS

16

Even people who love their long locks may sometimes yearn for a shorter style. In this design, the hair is folded inward and upward to create a surprising cropped look.

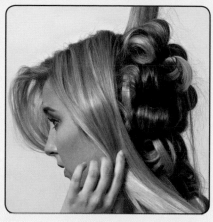

1

1. Wash and blow dry the hair. Mist the hair with holding spray. Starting at the back of the head, gather 1-inch sections of hair and curl them with a medium curling iron.

2. Backcomb each section before curling it, for maximum volume.

3. Place the curling iron as close to the root as possible for maximum volume.

4. Make a side part from the brow to the crown, and continue curling sections of hair at the front of the head.

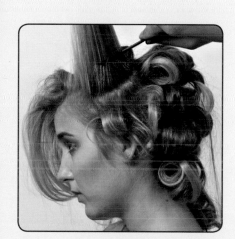

2

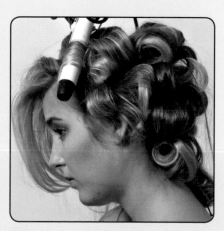

3

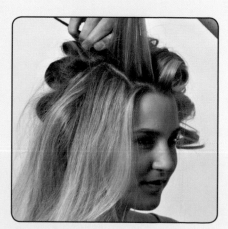

4

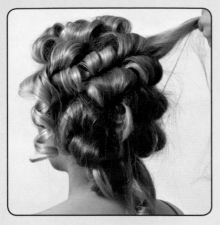

5

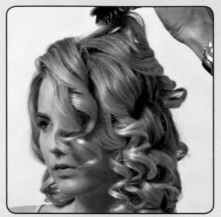

6

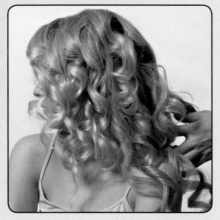

7

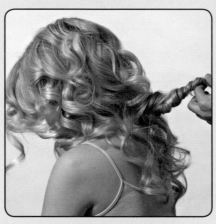

8

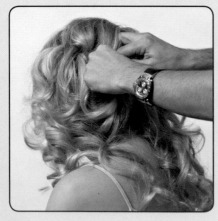

9

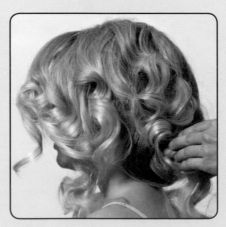

10

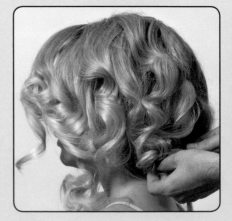

11

5. Curl all of the hair with the curling iron. Mist it with holding spray, and wait about 10 minutes for it to set.

6. Gently brush out the curls, to loosen them and create gentle waves.

7. Brush out all the curls, taking care not to brush away the wave.

8. Grasp a lock of hair at the ends and twist it gently.

9. Fold the twisted lock and secure it under the hair at the back of the head with a bobby pin.

10. Continue twisting locks of hair, folding them, and securing them under the head.

11. Try to fold all locks of hair evenly all around the head.

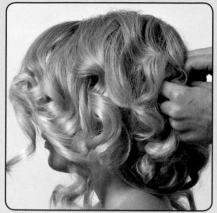

12

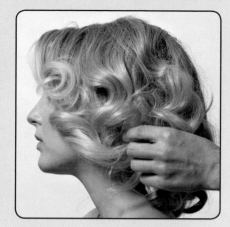

13

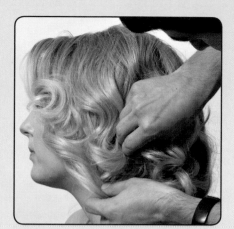

14

12. Leave the hair at the front of the head loose as you secure the hair all around the head.

13. Gently draw back the loose hair at the front of the head, pinning it carefully so as not to damage the curls.

14. Pin back the front hair to give an even, shoulder-length look all around the head.

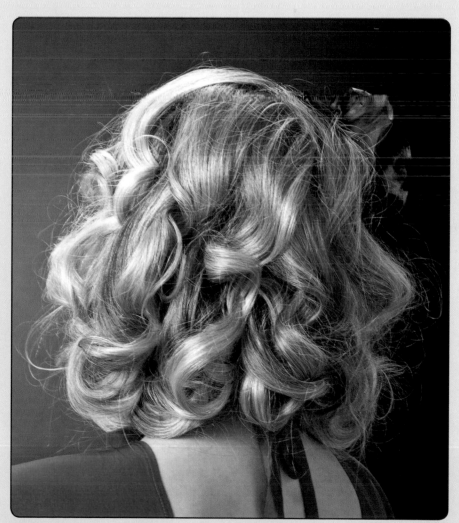

15

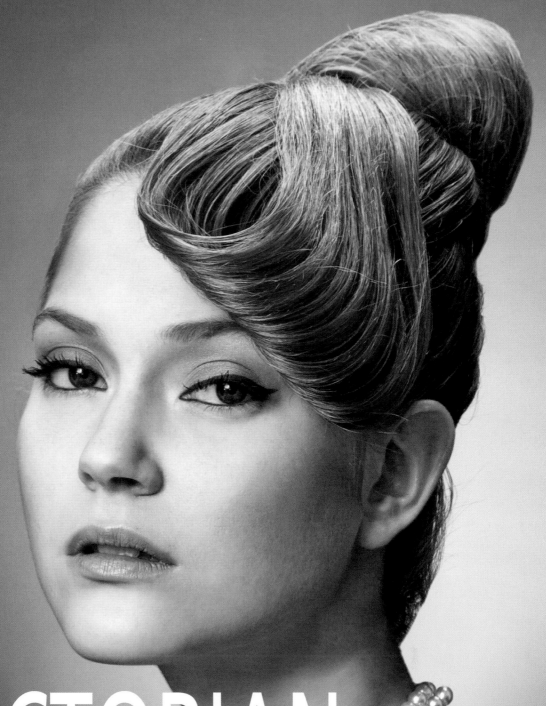

VICTORIAN

FOLDED LOOPS

17

This style is a fusion of Victorian elegance and modern ease. The hair at the back is drawn into a cone-shaped bun; at the front, it loops into a gentle fold.

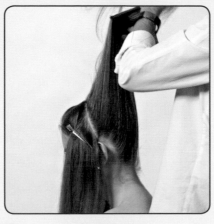

1

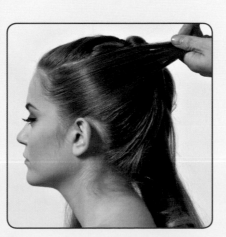

2

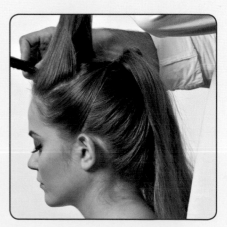

3

4

1. Wash and blow dry the hair. Make a part that extends from the top of each ear over the crown of the head, and gather the hair below the part, brushing it upward.

2. Bring the twisted hair upward to create a banana shape at the back of the head, and secure it with a clip.

3. Divide the hair at the front of the head into three sections. Gather the side sections together at the back of the head into a ponytail. Mist the hair with holding spray.

4. Brush the middle section of hair at the brow upward.

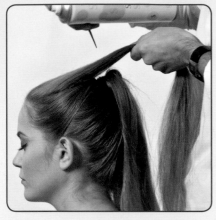

5

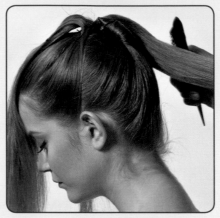

6

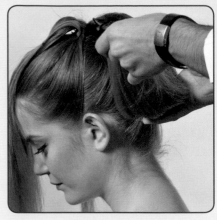

7

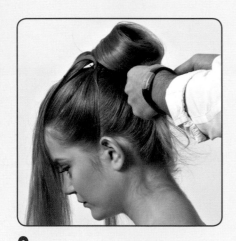

8

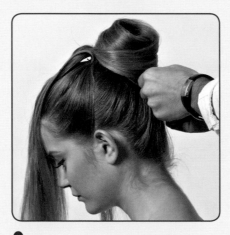

9

5. Mist the hair with holding spray and draw the hair backward. Secure the hair at the top of the ponytail with a clip.

6. Gently separate the lower part of the hair from the ponytail.

7. Wrap the hair in a loop around the base of the ponytail.

8. Continue wrapping the bottom of the hair around the base to form a high bun.

9. Tuck the ends of the hair under the bun, and secure the bun with bobby pins near the roots.

10. Mist the bun with holding spray and smooth the surface with the back of a comb.

11. Comb out the section of hair at the front of the bun.

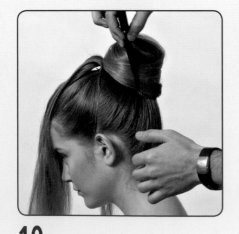

10

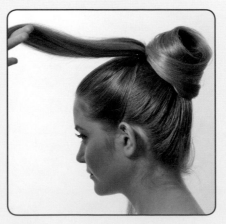

11

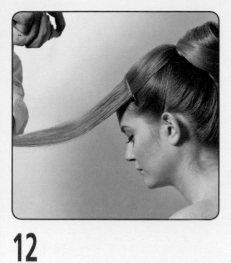

12

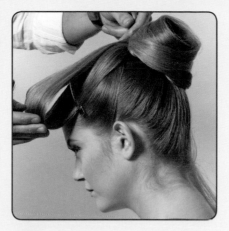

13

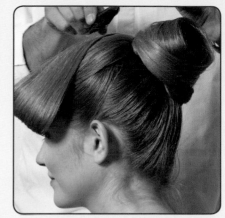

14

12. Brush the hair forward and secure it at one side of the head, near the brow. Mist the ends with holding spray.

13. Fold this section of hair backward, bringing it over the crown of the head and drawing the ends to the bun.

14. Secure the ends at the top center of the bun with bobby pins. Smooth the hair with the back of a comb, and mist with holding spray.

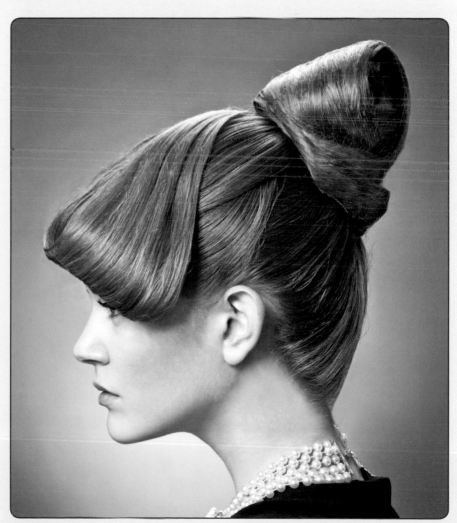

15

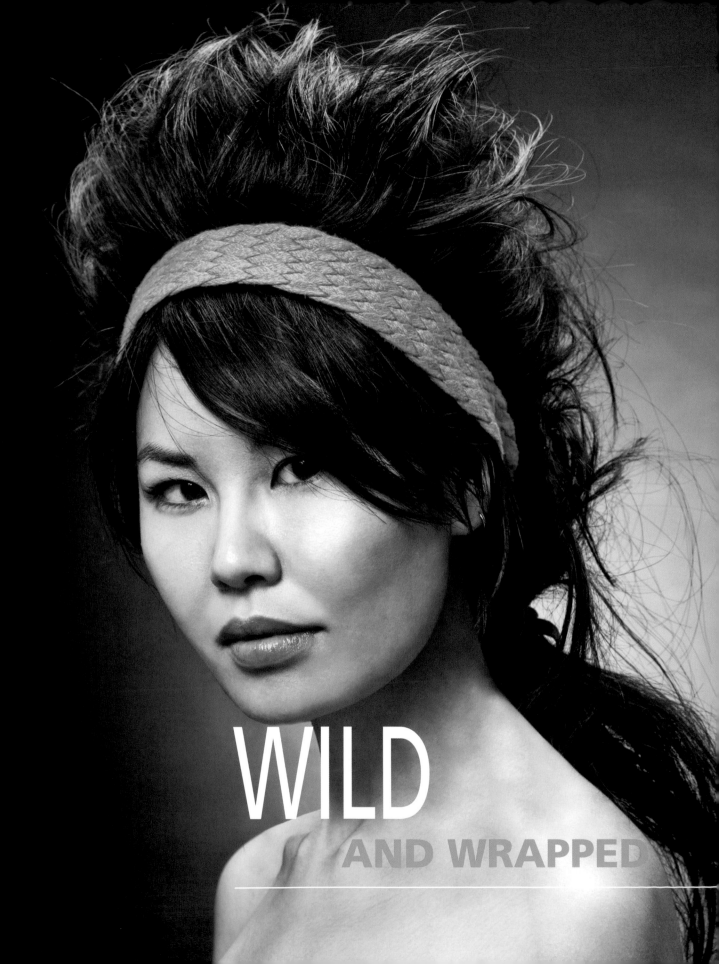

WILD

AND WRAPPED

18

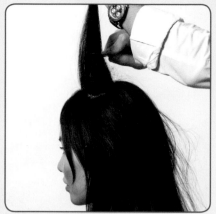

1

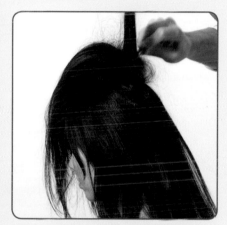

2

This high hairstyle features a wild-looking extra-thick ponytail at the back. The bangs hang playfully to one side, and a hair band adds a bright strip of color.

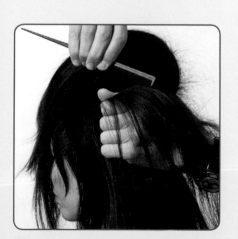

3

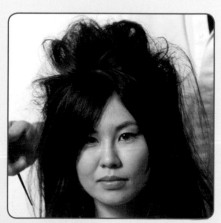

4

1. Wash and blow dry the hair. Gather a 1 x 1½-inch section of hair at the top of the crown, just behind the bangs. Hold it upward at the ends, and backcomb it to the roots.

2. Gather a similar section of hair from behind the first section, and backcomb it to the roots. Repeat this process all the way down the middle of the head, from just behind the bangs to the nape of the neck.

3. Backcomb similar sections of hair to the right and left of the crown.

4. Bring the backcombed hair backward, arranging it to keep maximum volume. Leave the hair at the front of the head loose.

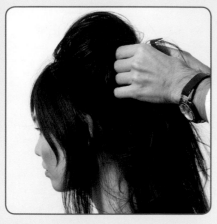

5

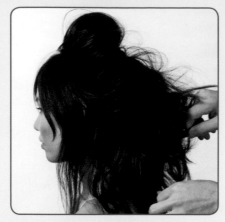

6

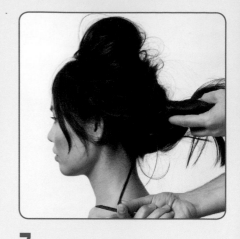

7

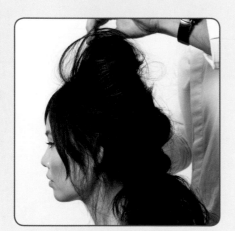

8

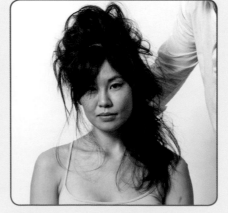

9

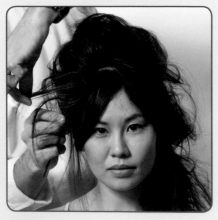

10

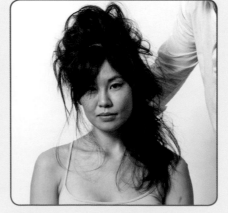

11

5. Gently brush back the backcombed hair, without reducing the volume, and gather it together at the back of the head, just below the crown. Secure it with bobby pins.

6. Backcomb sections of hair at the back of the head to create a wild-looking high-volume look.

7. Gather the hair at the back of the head, and twist it into a thick coil. Pin the coil to the head with bobby pins, leaving the ends loose.

8. Mist the hair with holding spray, and selectively loosen strands from the lifted hair at the front.

9. Backcomb the loose hair ends near the nape of the neck.

10. Backcomb the hair along the brow to increase volume. Arrange the ends of hair from the back over one shoulder.

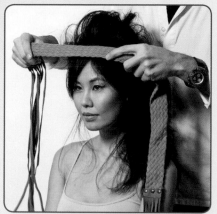

12

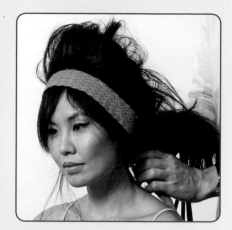

13

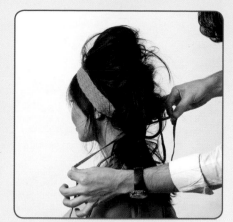

14

11. Adjust hair to create a stylishly relaxed look.

12. Select a brightly colored headband and position it around the head, just above the hairline.

13. Arrange the headband so that it lies over the bangs at the front of the head, but below the hair at the nape of the neck.

14. Tie the headband at the nape of the neck and use it to gather the loose hair, as desired.

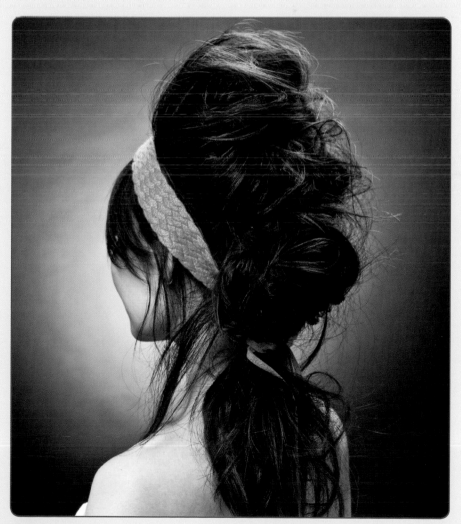

15

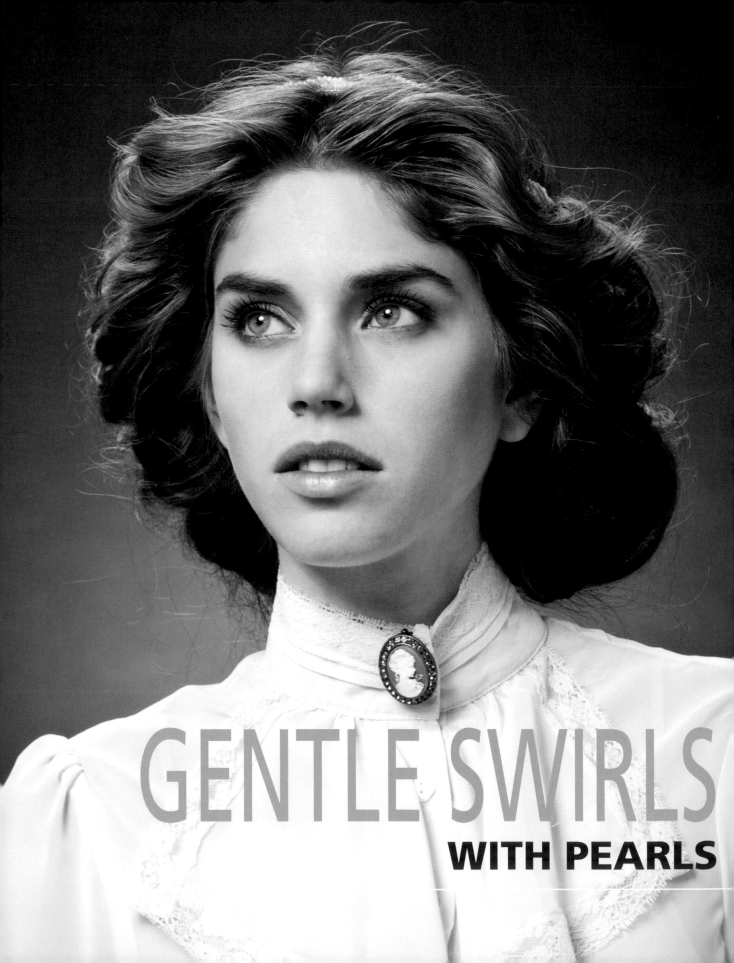

GENTLE SWIRLS
WITH PEARLS

19

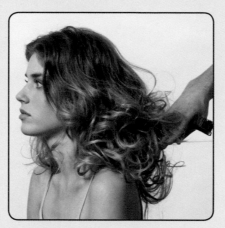

1

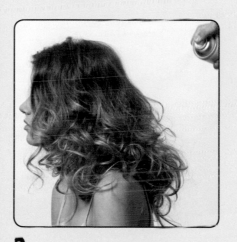

2

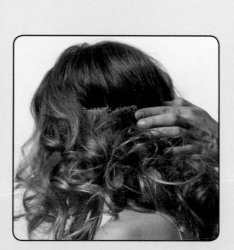

3

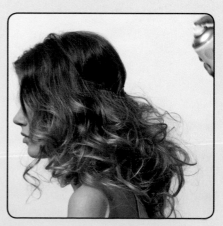

4

1. Wash and blow dry the hair. Curl it with a medium curling iron to add body. Backcomb the hair ends with your fingers to add volume.

2. Mist the hair with holding spray.

3. Insert bobby pins in a semi-circle around the back of the head at the base of the crown.

4. Mist the hair again with holding spray. Make sure the bobby pins are tightly secured, enough to hold the hair that will soon be folded up to them.

This classic design is soft, subtle, and very feminine. Upgrade it with a strand of folded pearls draped delicately at the back.

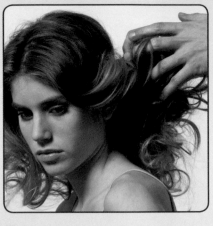

5

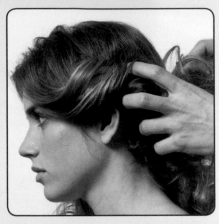

6

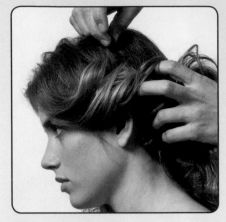

7

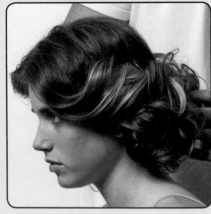

8

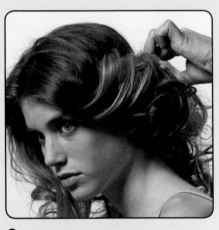

9

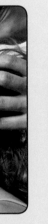

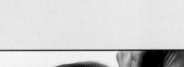

5. Draw up the hair at one side of the face and roll it into a very loose roll, upward and toward the back of the head.

6. Roll the hair toward the row of bobby pins. Use your hands, rather than a comb, to avoid damaging the curls.

7. Secure the rolled hair with the bobby pins already in place, and add additional bobby pins as necessary.

8. Repeat with another section of hair, moving your way toward the back of the head and rolling it upward in the same manner.

9. Continue affixing rolled sections of hair to the line of bobby pins until you reach the back of the head.

10. Repeat the process on the other side of the head, starting at the front and working your way toward the back. Make sure

10

11

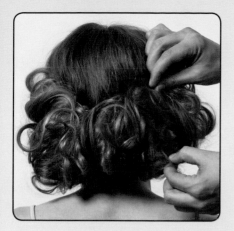

12

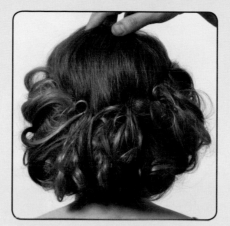

13

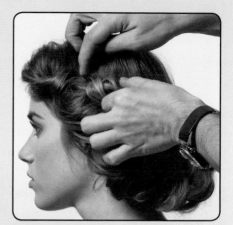

14

to keep the rolled hair looking loose and natural.

11. Use bobby pins to secure the rolled hair, and mist the hair with holding spray to secure.

12. Gently loosen some of the locks to create a full and luscious look all around the head.

13. Arrange the rolled sections of hair so that there are arranged in an even line all around the crown.

14. Secure the hairstyle with bobby pins as required, and mist it with holding spray.

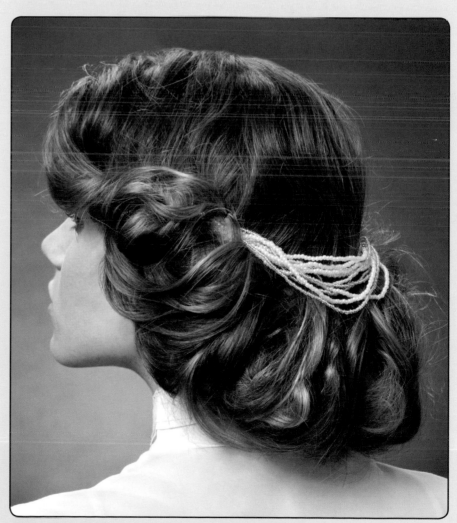

15

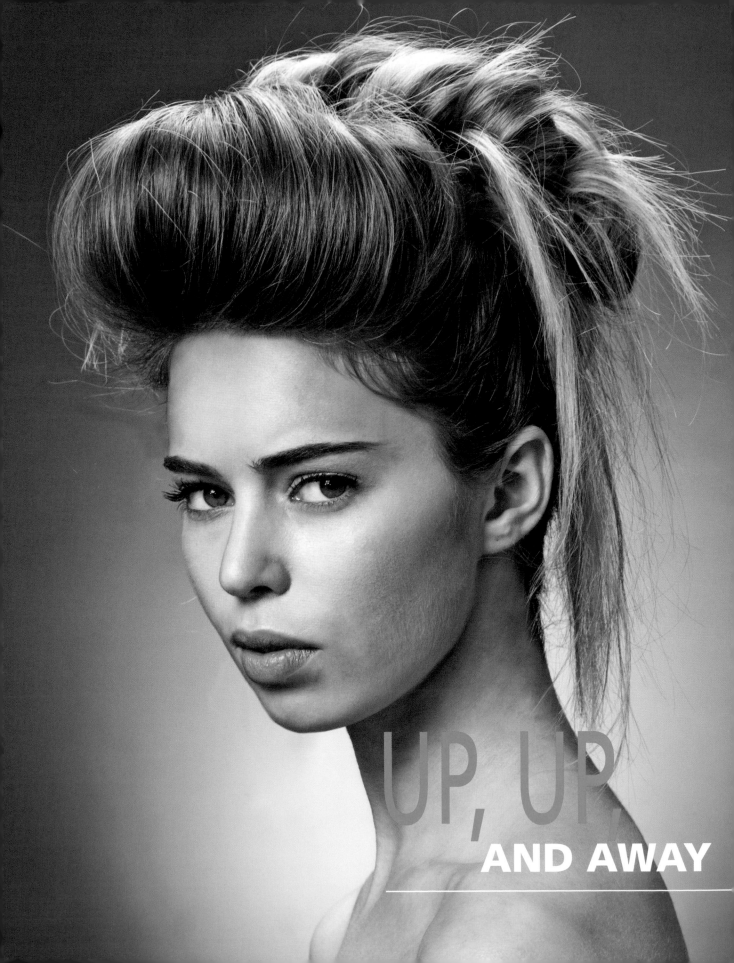

UP, UP

AND AWAY

20

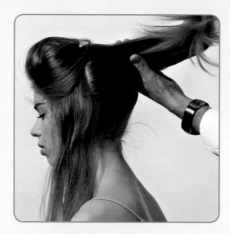

1

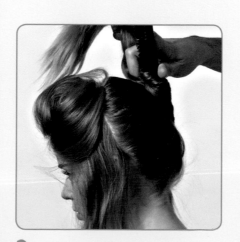

2

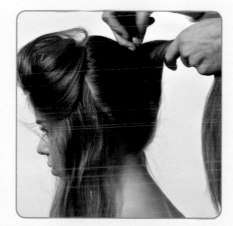

3

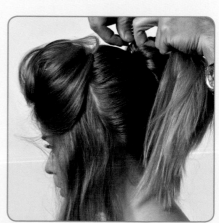

4

1. Wash and blow dry the hair. Make a part that extends from behind each ear over the crown of the head, and gather the hair below the part.

2. Draw up the hair at the back of the head, twisting it gently.

3. Bring the twisted hair upward to create a banana shape at the back of the head.

4. Secure the twisted hair to the head, just above the banana shape, with bobby pins.

This extra high hairstyle accentuates the face thanks to the highly swept bangs. The back of the hairstyle features a loosely knotted bun and random loose strands of hair.

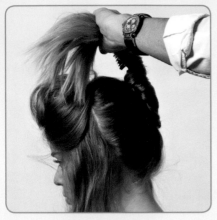

5

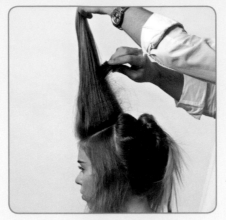

6

5. Continue twisting the hair, allowing it to form a U-shape. Pin the rolled hair to the head, leaving the ends loose.

6. Divide the hair in front of the part into three sections and backcomb the middle section.

7. Mist the backcombed hair with holding spray.

8. Secure the ends of this section with an elastic band.

9. Fold this section of hair backward and bring the elastic band toward the roots to create a high wave at the brow. Secure the hair near the elastic band to the head with bobby pins.

10. Comb the hair at the sides of the head upward and backward.

11. Mist the hair lightly with holding spray; then comb the hair upward and backward.

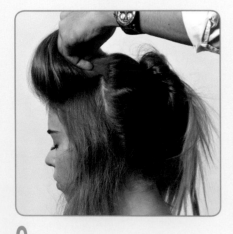

7

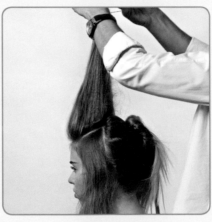

8

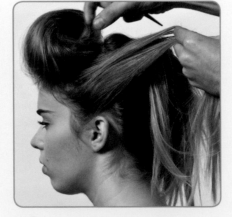

9

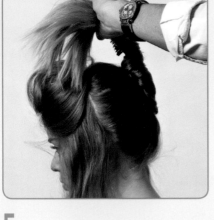

10

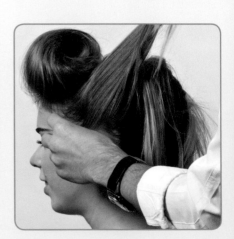

11

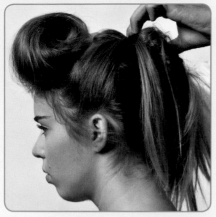

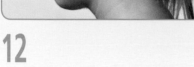

12

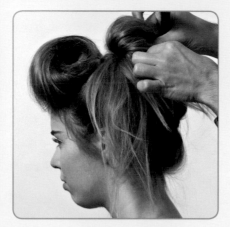

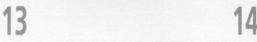

13

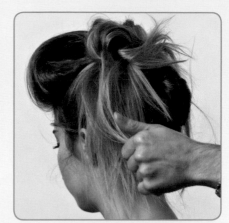

14

12. Secure the hair at the base of the twisted bun, below the crown.

13. Twist the loose ends of hair around the bun to create extra volume.

14. Style the ends so that they are evenly spaced and fan out around the bun. Mist the hair with holding spray.

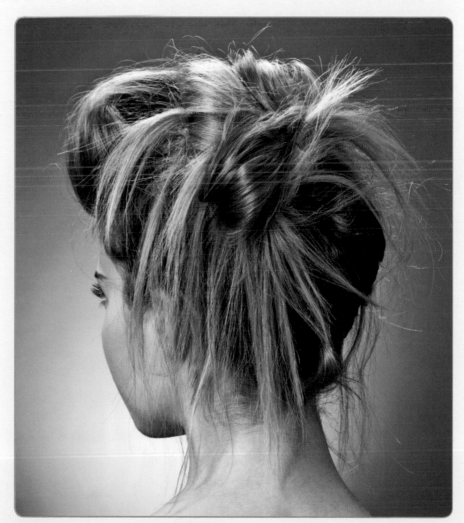

15

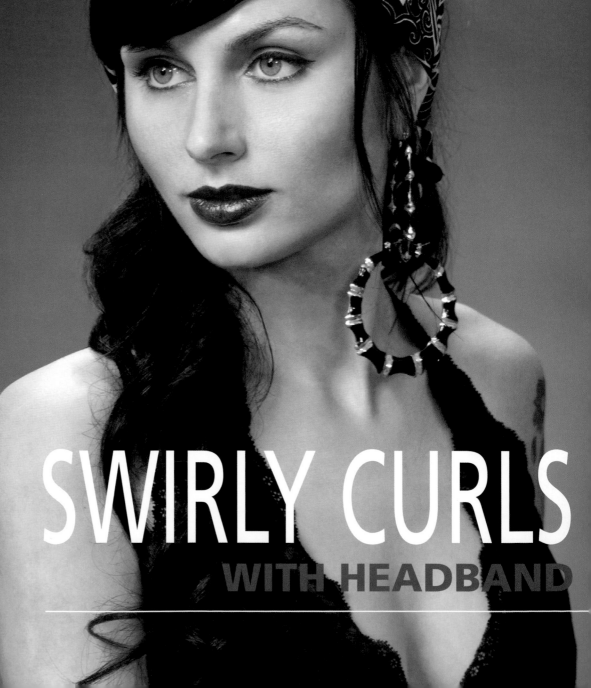

SWIRLY CURLS
WITH HEADBAND

21

This long, curly style adds length and gentle curls to your hair. Tie it up with a colorful headband for a bright and fun finish.

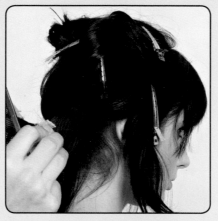

1

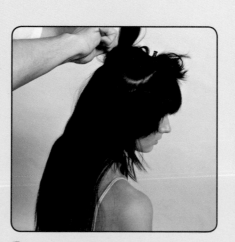

2

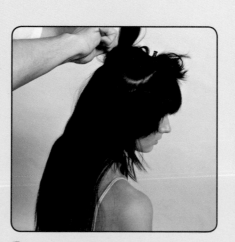

3

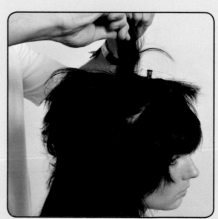

4

1. Wash and blow dry the hair straight. Make a part that extends from behind each ear across the back of the head. Secure the hair above the part. Backcomb the hair below the part, from the end of the hair toward the root.

2. Select a hair extension that matches the color of the hair. Attach it close to the roots of the backcombed hair for a strong and lasting grip.

3. Gather a lock of hair from the crown and backcomb.

4. Gather and backcomb a lock of hair 2 inches across by 1 inch down starting 3 inches from the brow.

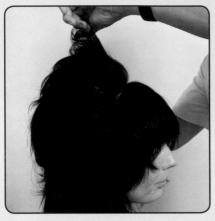

5

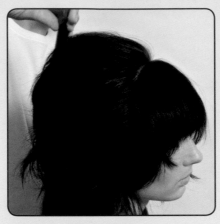

6

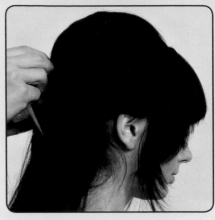

7

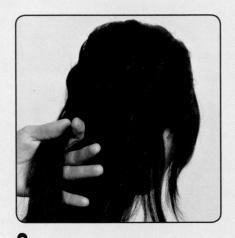

8

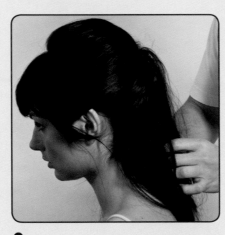
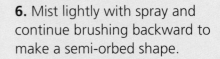
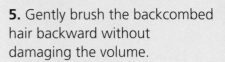

9

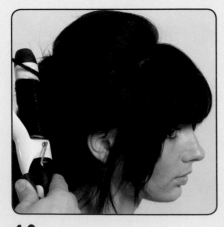

10

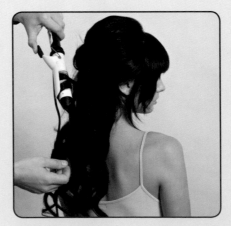
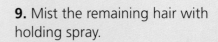

11

5. Gently brush the backcombed hair backward without damaging the volume.

6. Mist lightly with spray and continue brushing backward to make a semi-orbed shape.

7. Gather the hair ends together at the back of the head and secure them in place with bobby pins.

8. Draw a small lock of hair from either side of the face and pin down each lock at the back of the head, near the center of the orb.

9. Mist the remaining hair with holding spray.

10. Gather a 2-inch wide lock from the remaining loose hair and curl it with a medium curling iron.

11. Continue curling the remaining loose hair in this manner.

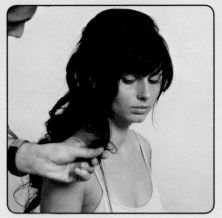

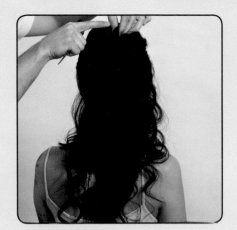

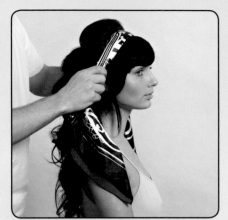

12

13

14

12. Hold the hair by the end and gently push the lock toward the root with your fingers.

13. Gather several strands of long hair from the back and fold them toward the crown to create a layered effect. Secure them at the base of the orb with bobby pins.

14. To complete the look, place a 1½-inch wide headband over the crown of the head, and tie at the nape of the neck below the hair.

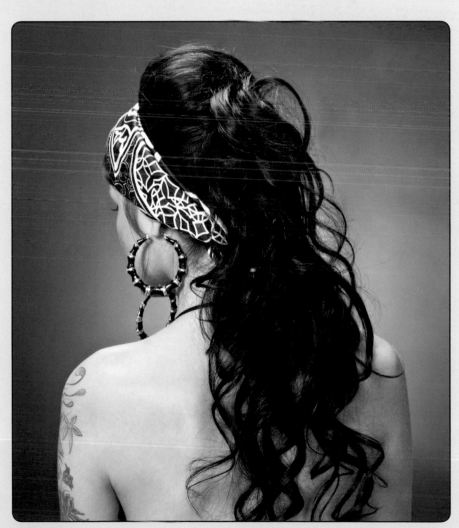

15

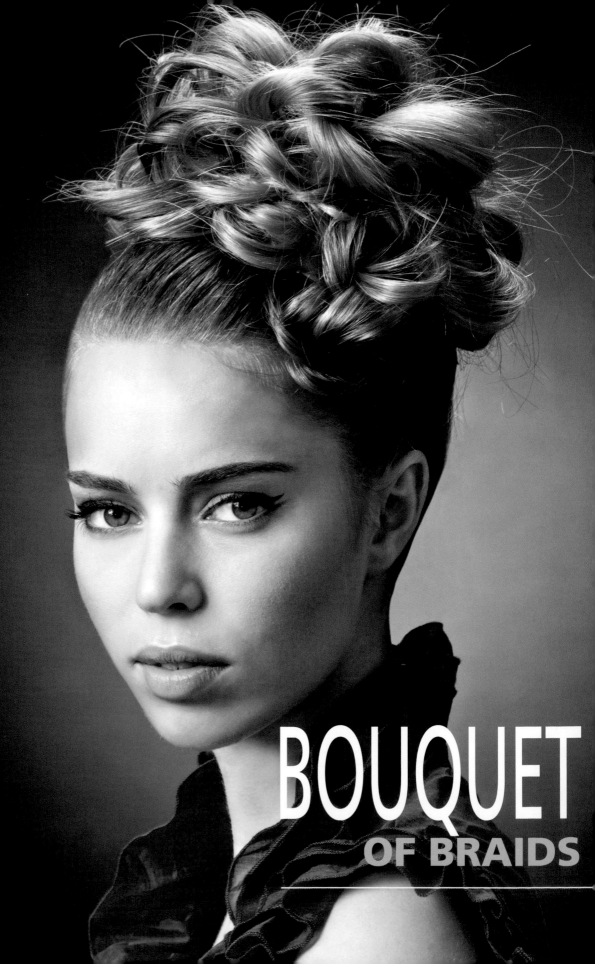

BOUQUET
OF BRAIDS

22

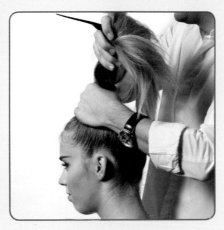

1. Wash and blow dry the hair. Gather the hair into a high ponytail at the top of the crown.

2. Secure the ponytail with an elastic band.

3. Divide the ponytail into six even sections.

4. Apply molding wax to each section.

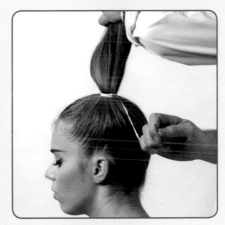

This fun hairstyle is made up of several loosened braids, gathered on the top of the head. Dramatic and fun, this hairstyle is deceptively simple to achieve.

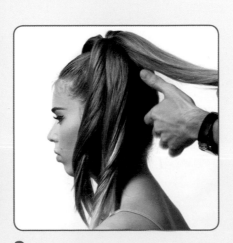

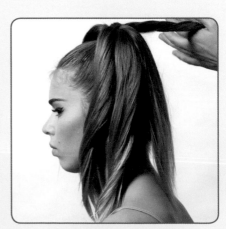

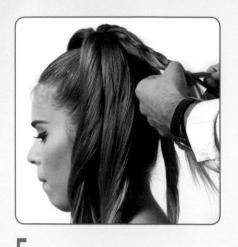

5

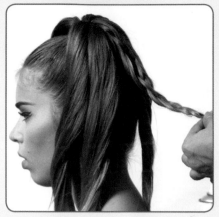

6

5. Divide one section of hair into three even sections. Braid the section into a loose braid.

6. Secure the end of the braid with an elastic band.

7. Repeat this process with the five remaining sections of hair.

8. Check that braids are loose by inserting your fingers in them.

9. Hold one braid by the ends.

10. Bring the braided hair toward the base of the ponytail; then fold the hair and secure the ends to the head near the base of the ponytail with bobby pins.

11. Repeat this process with the five remaining braids.

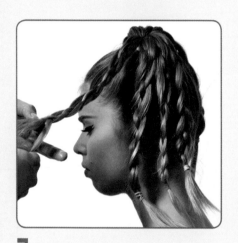

7

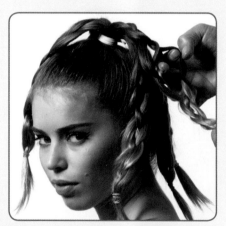

8

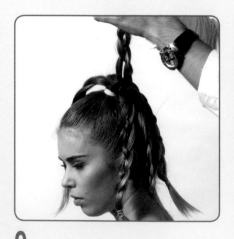

9

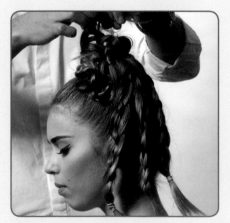

10

11

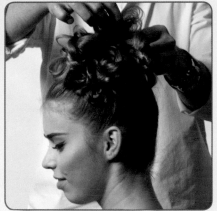

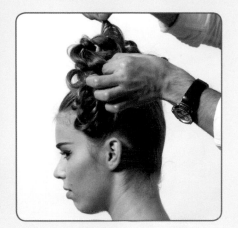

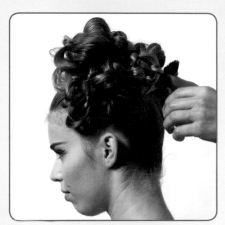

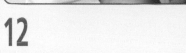

12

13

14

12. Once all the braids have been gathered and the ends secured, tug gently on several locks in each braid to loosen them.

13. Arrange the loosened locks as desired.

14. Comb up the hair at the top and back of the head, and mist with holding spray to finish.

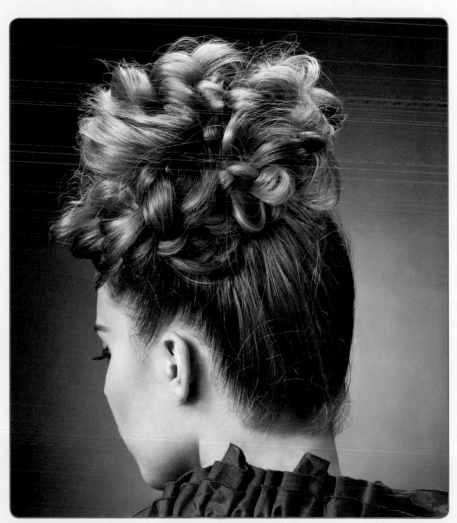

15

WAVES
TO THE WAIST

23

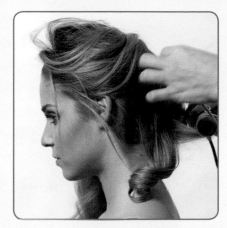

1

1. Wash and blow dry the hair. Divide the hair into 1-inch sections and curl the sections with a medium curling iron, starting at the nape of the neck and moving upward. Backcomb each section of hair before curling, for maximum volume.

2. After each section has been curled, secure the curls with bobby pins and mist them with holding spray.

3. Continue curling 1-inch sections of hair at the top of the head as well, and secure with bobby pins.

4. Curl the hair at the brow.

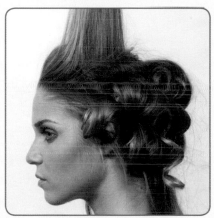

2

Show off naturally long hair with this pretty style. The front hair is voluminous, with gentle curls for balance at the back. The rest of the hair is lovely and loose.

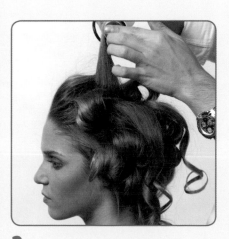

3

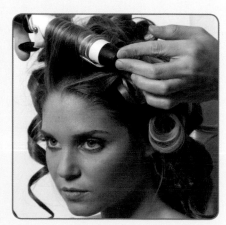

4

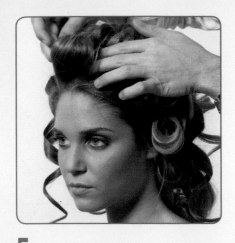

5

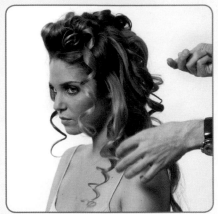

6

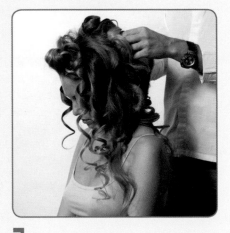

7

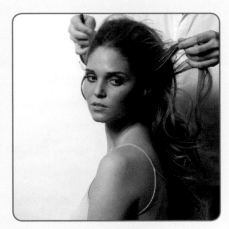

8

5. Secure the curls with bobby pins, mist them with holding spray, and wait for about 10 minutes for the curls set.

6. Gently release the curls by removing the bobby pins and loosing the curls with your fingers.

7. Once all the curls have been released, mist the hair with holding spray.

8. Run your fingers through the curls gently, to open them.

9. Draw the hair at the sides and front of the head backward, and secure it at the back of the head with bobby pins.

10. Arrange the pinned hair so that it blends naturally with the rest of the hair at the back of the head.

11. Roll a small lock of hair at the back of the head into a loop, and secure it with a bobby pin.

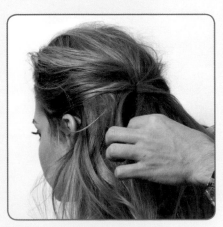

9

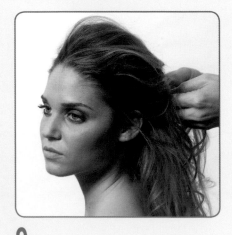

10

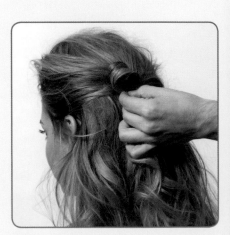

11

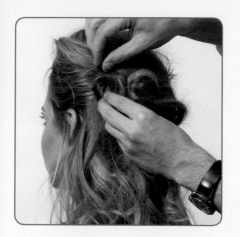

12

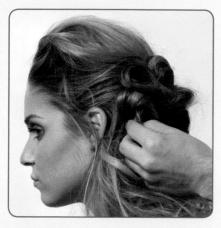

13

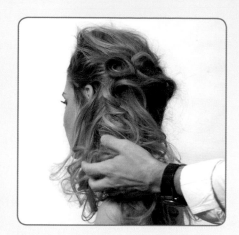

14

12. Repeat on the other side by looping another lock of hair at the back of the head and securing it with bobby pins.

13. Make a couple more loops of hair below the first two loops, and secure them with bobby pins.

14. Arrange the loose hair by letting it hang at the back or bringing it forward over one shoulder. Mist the hair with holding spray.

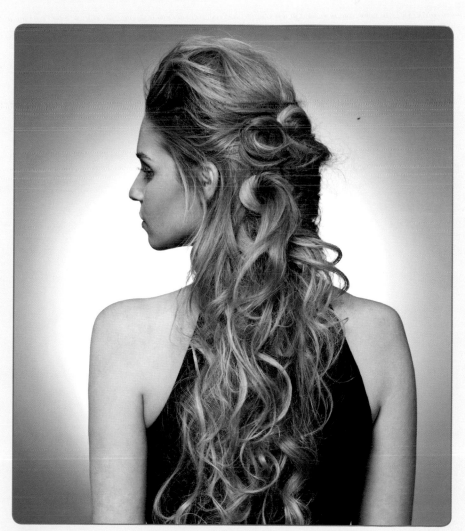

15

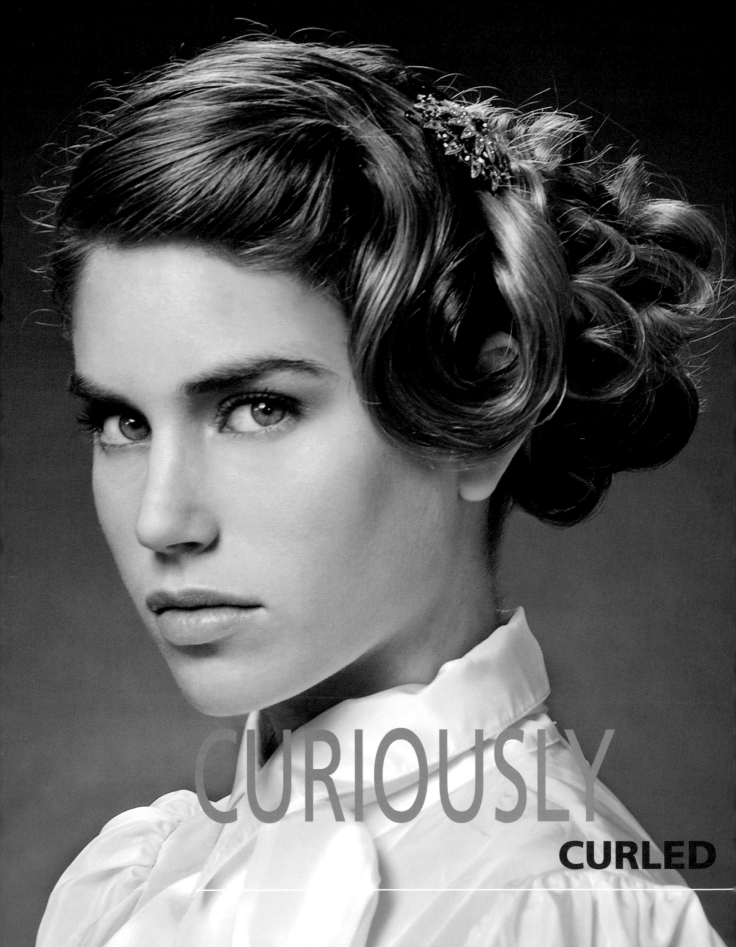

CURIOUSLY

CURLED

24

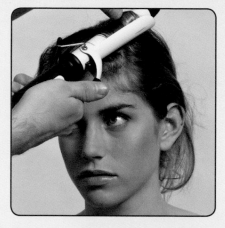

1

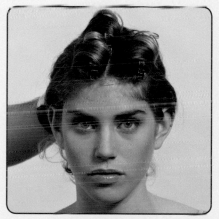

2

This look features a luscious collection of curls, all of which are gathered gently behind one ear. A single lock falls gracefully to one side of the face, softening the look.

1. Wash and blow dry the hair. Divide the hair at the brow into three even sections, and curl the middle section of hair with a medium curling iron.

2. Make two side-by-side curls at the top of the head. Secure with clips and mist with holding spray.

3. Make a part that extends from the top of each ear over the crown. Gather the hair below the part into a ponytail and mist with holding spray. Hold the hair in front of the part with clips.

4. Draw out a lock at the top of the ponytail and roll it into a double loop. Secure the ponytail with a bobby pin above the base. Repeat this process with more locks of hair at the top of the ponytail.

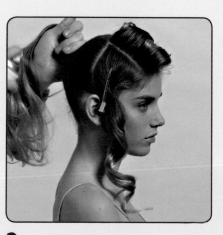

3

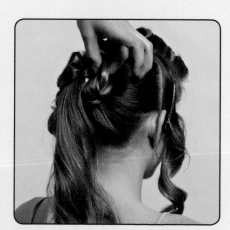

4

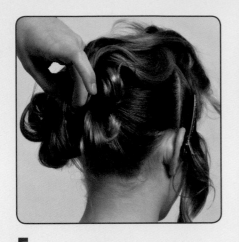

5

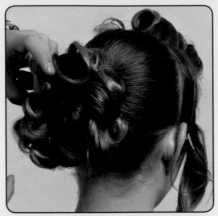
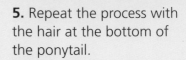
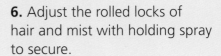

6

5. Repeat the process with the hair at the bottom of the ponytail.

6. Adjust the rolled locks of hair and mist with holding spray to secure.

7. Twist one of the loose sections of hair at the front of the head, drawing it backward behind the ear.

8. Secure this section near the base of the ponytail. Roll the ends into a double loop and secure it as well.

9. Remove the clips from the curls at the front of the head, and gently open up the curls.

10. Comb the hair gently to create waves.

11. Draw the waved hair backward and to one side, shaping it to maintain volume. Secure it with a clip.

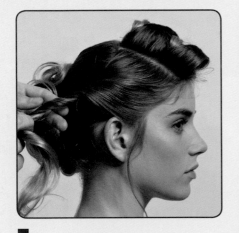

7

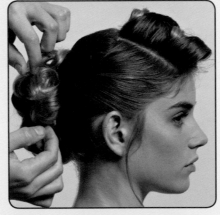

8

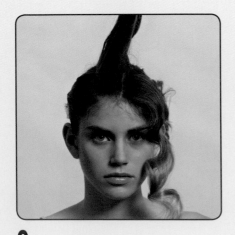

9

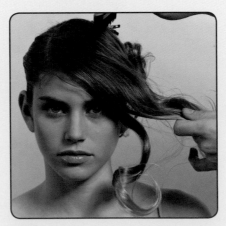

10

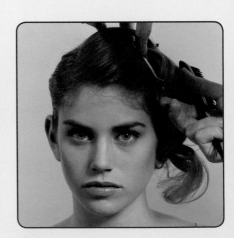

11

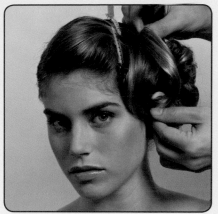

12

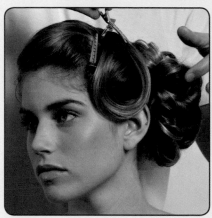

13

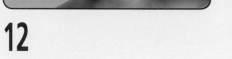

14

12. Comb the hair below the clip, styling it into gentle waves, and secure it with clips.

13. Style the hair gently at this point since it isn't yet firmly secured.

14. Once all the hair is secured, mist it with holding spray and dry it with a diffuser. When the hairstyle is in place, remove the clips and add a hair accessory.

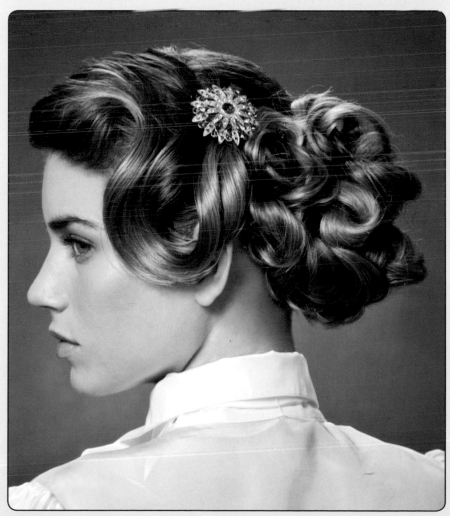

15

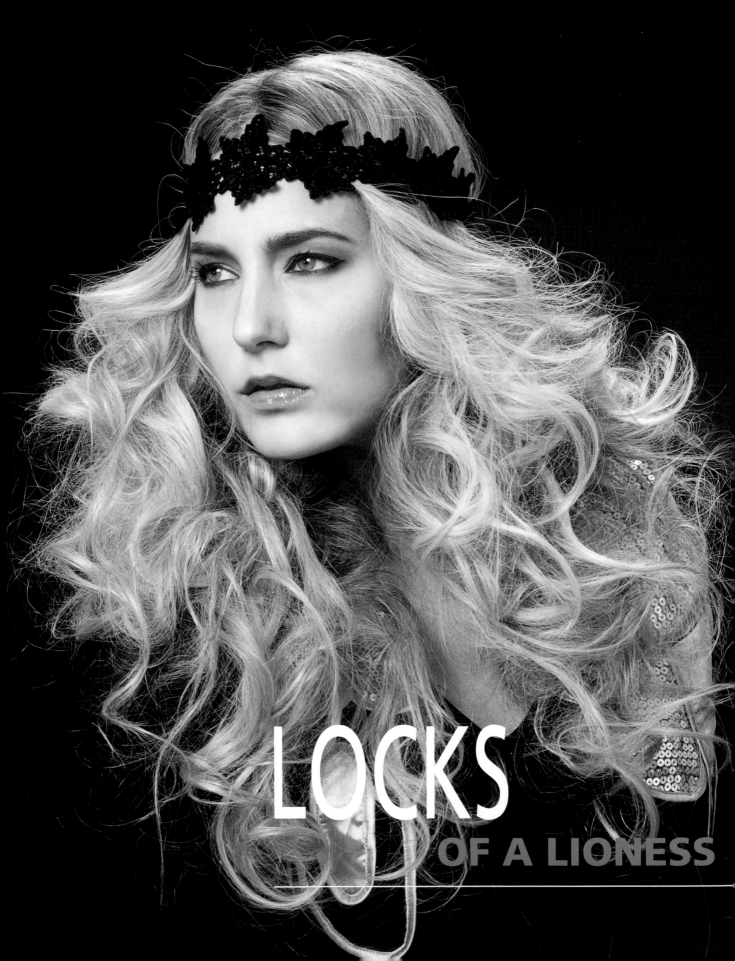

LOCKS
OF A LIONESS

25

The bottom of this hairstyle has plenty of volume thanks to a heavy dose of bold, beautiful waves. The smoothed down top offers a striking contrast that is accented by a sequined hair band.

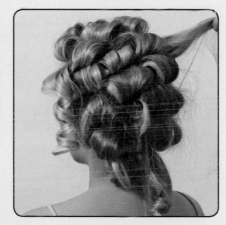

1

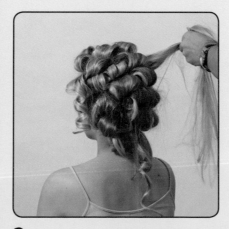

2

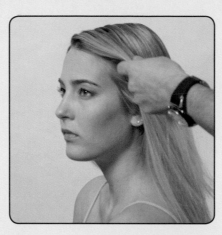

3

1. Wash and blow dry the hair straight.

2. Curl the entire head of hair, section by section, with a medium curling iron.

3. Release the hair from the curlers.

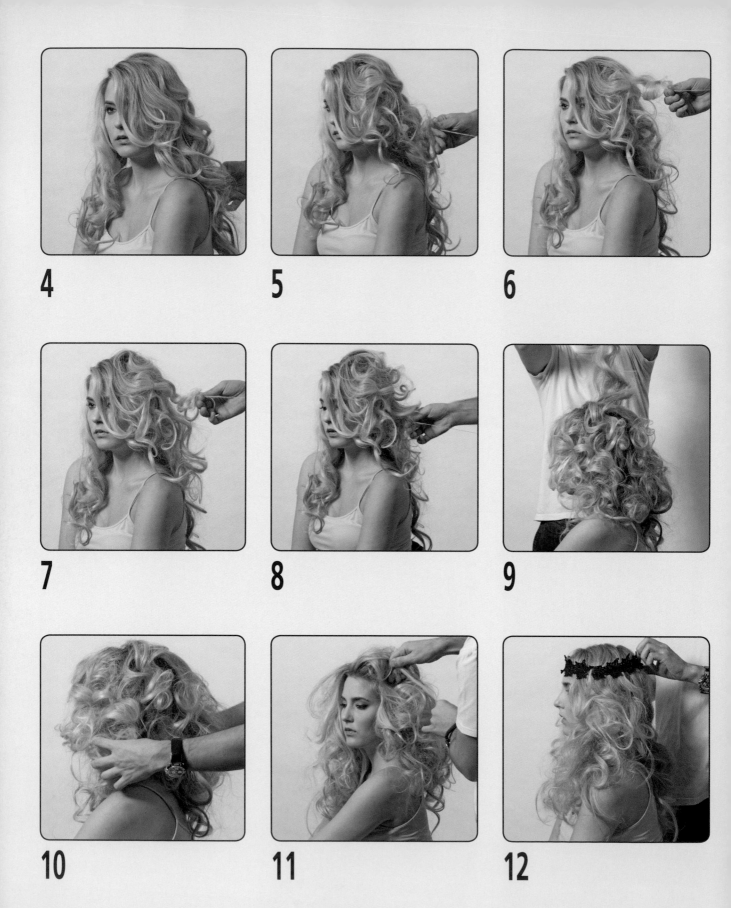

4

5

6

7

8

9

10

11

12

4. Run your fingers through the curls to open them up and create a wavy look.

5. Grasp a small lock of hair with one hand, and draw the hand upward, from the ends to the root, to backcomb the hair.

6. Continue backcombing the curls at the back of the head.

7. The hair will start looking full and extravagant.

8. Mist the hair occasionally with holding spray to preserve the volume.

9. Backcomb the curls at the crown too, to continue increasing volume.

10. Apply molding wax by rubbing a bit between your hands and then scrunching the hair all around.

11. Backcomb the hair a bit more, to increase volume as desired and create a voluptuous, carefree look.

12. Flatten the hair at the top, and secure a band around the crown.

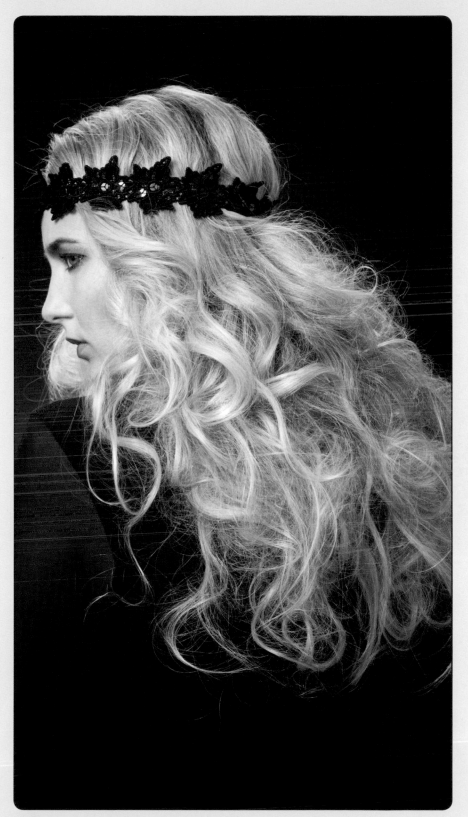

13

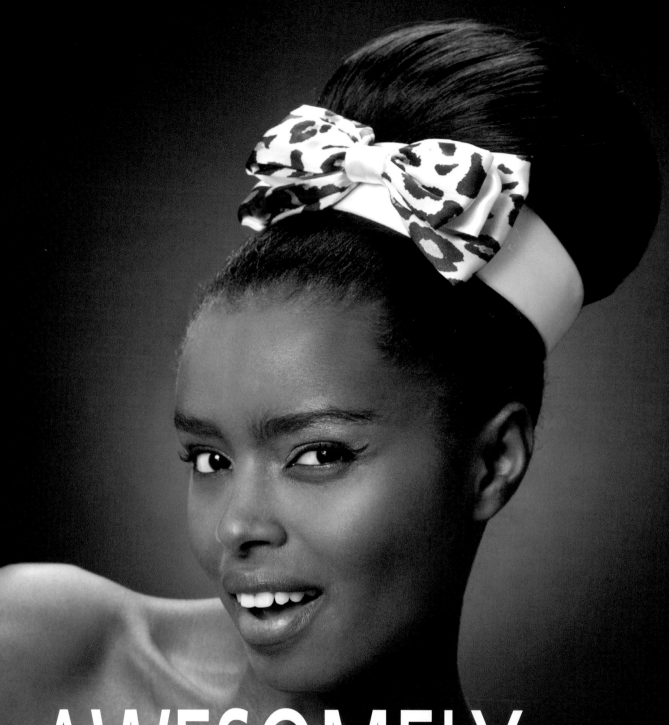

AWESOMELY

OVERSIZED BUN

26

The oversized bun in this design is set high on the head and won't go unnoticed. Just to make sure this hairstyle attracts attention, add a leopard-print bow for effect.

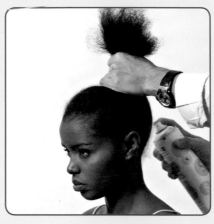

1

1. Wash and blow dry the hair. Gather the hair in a high ponytail and mist it with holding spray.

2. For maximum smoothness all around, comb the hair upward while blow drying, and mist with holding spray to secure.

3. Select hair extensions that match the color of the hair.

4. Affix the extensions around the base of the ponytail.

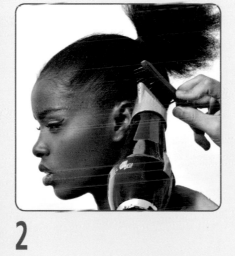

2

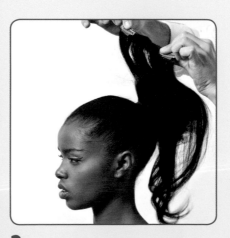

3

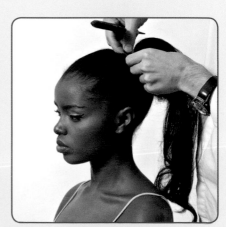

4

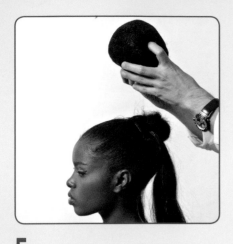

5

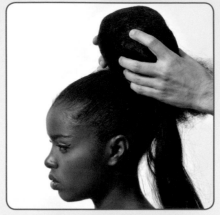

6

5. Select a sponge that matches the color of the hair, and shape it into a ball.

6. Affix the sponge above the base of the ponytail with bobby pins.

7. Divide the loose hair into two sections on either side of the head. Comb one section upward, and arrange it over the sponge.

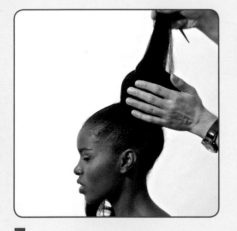

7

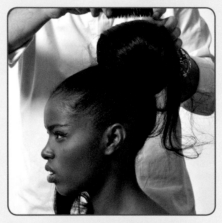

8

8. Brush the hair so that it covers the entire sponge.

9. Mist the hair with holding spray to secure it over the sponge.

10. Wrap the ends around the bun to create a smooth surface.

11. Pin the ends of the hair to the bun.

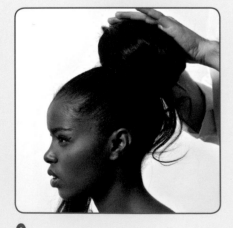

9

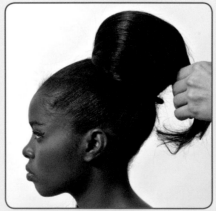

10

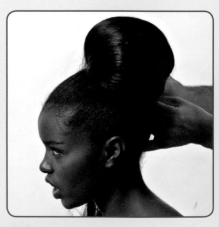

11

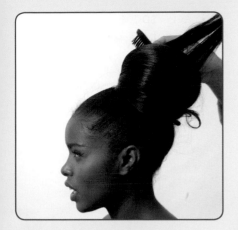

12

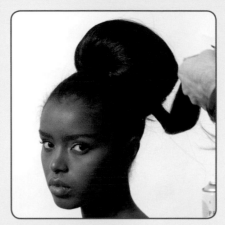

13

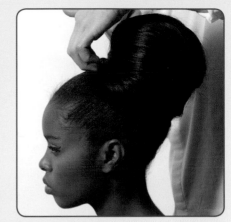

14

12. Brush the other section of hair and wrap it over the bun in the same direction. Secure the hair to the sponge with bobby pins.

13. Mist the loose ends of hair with holding spray; then comb it flat.

14. Wrap the hair around the base of the sponge like a ribbon, and secure it with bobby pins. Mist the hair with holding spray to secure.

15. To complete the look, wrap a hair band around the base of the bun.

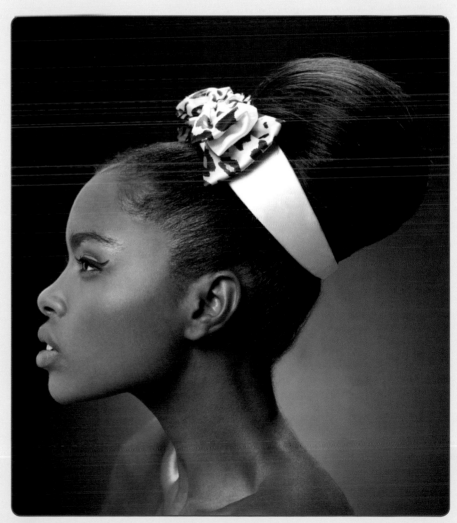

15

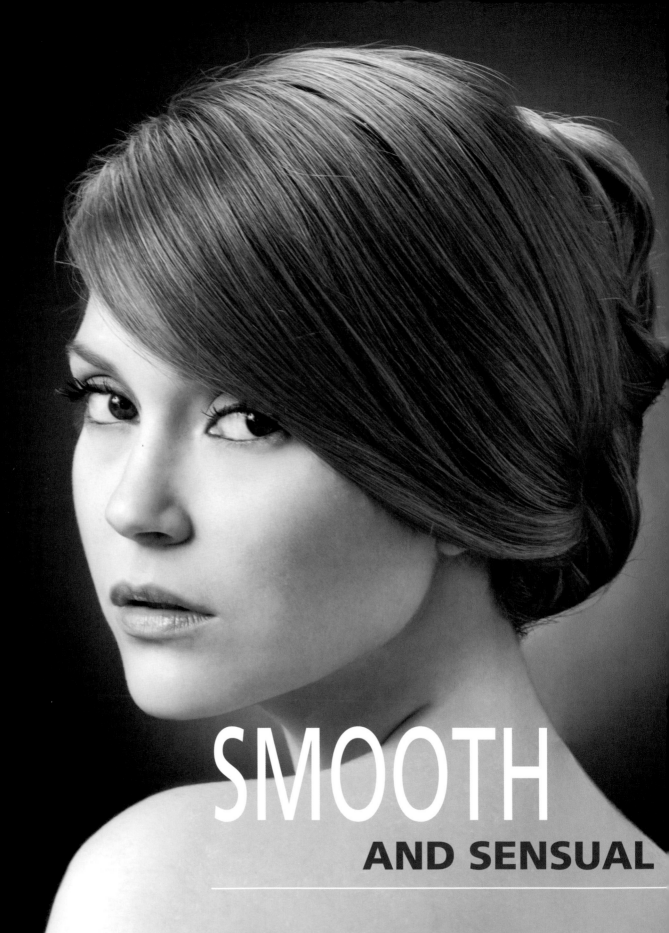

SMOOTH
AND SENSUAL

27

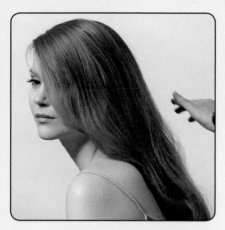

1. Wash and blow dry the hair straight.

2. Make a deep right side part and comb the hair above the part so that it hangs gently over the left brow.

3. Draw the hair toward the back of the head and downward. Secure at the nape of the neck, on the right side, with a clip.

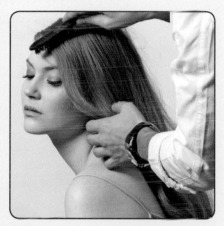

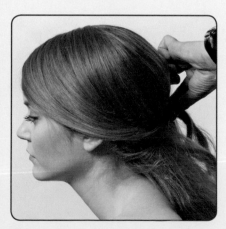

This hairstyle features an extreme side part, for a sensual, secretive look. At the back, the cone-shaped twist exposes a lovely bare neck.

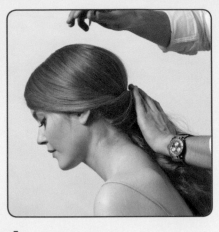

4

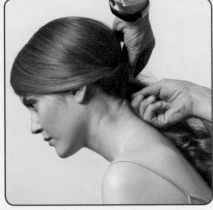

5

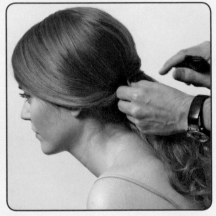

6

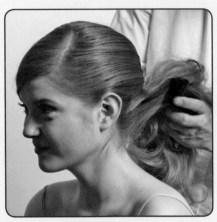

7

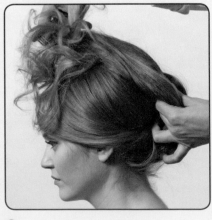

8

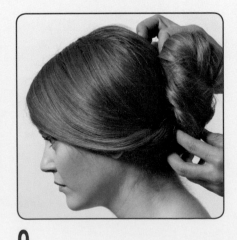

9

4. Brush the hair on the left side of the head upward and backward, toward the nape of the neck.

5. Secure the hair with a line of bobby pins at the nape of the neck, exposing the left side of the head, and gather the hair together.

6. Gather the hair from the right side of the head backward and upward, and secure it at the back of the head with a bobby pin.

7. Brush together the hair gathered at the back of the head.

8. Fold the hair upward and forward while twisting it.

9. Twist the hair around itself.

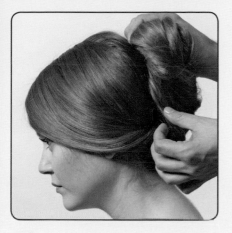

10

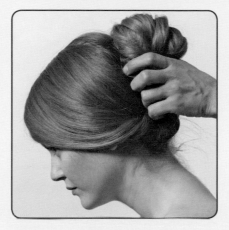

11

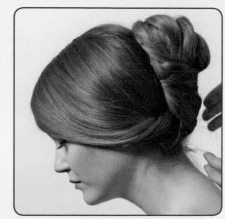

12

10. Secure the twisted hair with bobby pins. Make sure the twist remains somewhat loose.

11. Make a banana-shaped twist with the ends of the hair.

12. Secure the entire twist with bobby pins and mist it with holding spray to secure.

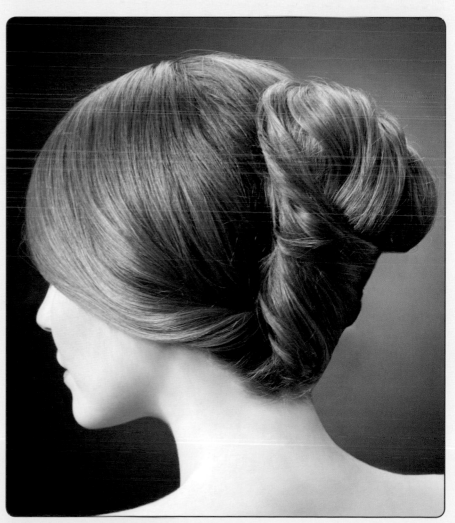

13

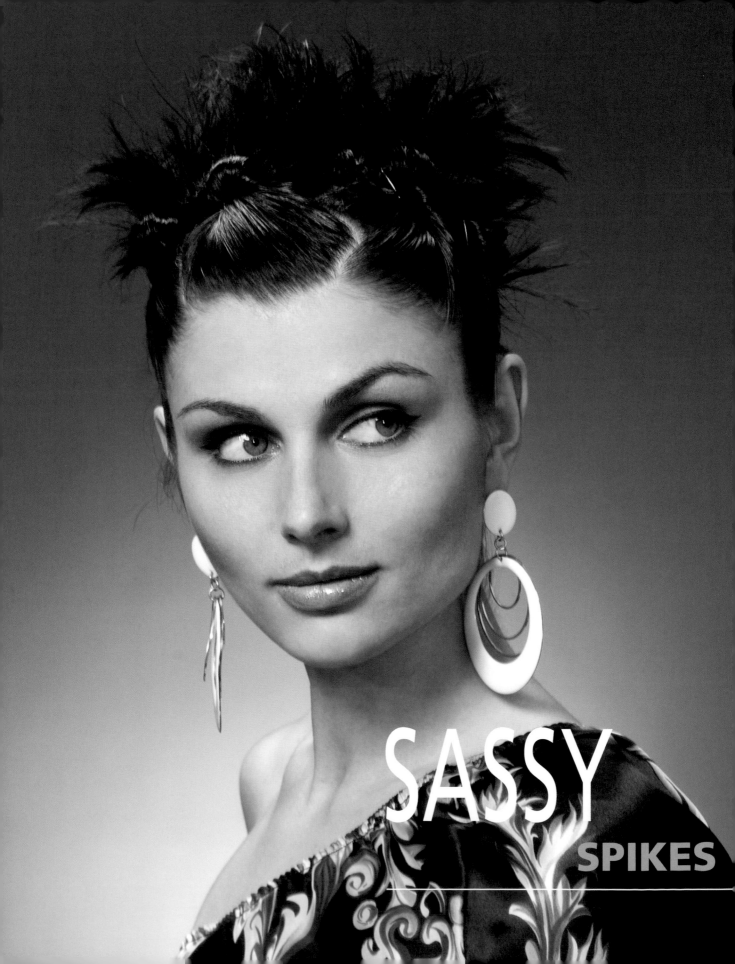

SASSY

SPIKES

28

This hairstyle has just the right combination of sassiness and style. With careful knots and carefree spikes, it will definitely turn heads.

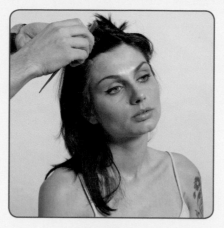

1

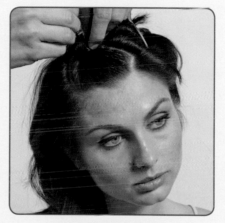

2

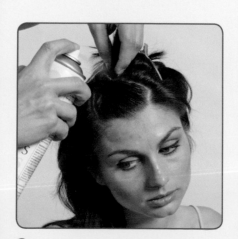

3

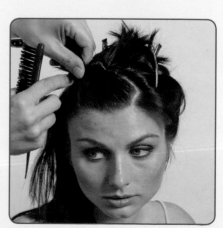

4

1. Wash and blow dry the hair. Divide the hair along the brow into small sections.

2. Comb each section backward and twist tightly along the roots to form a rope. Secure each rope with a bobby pin.

3. Position the holding spray close to the roots and mist the hair from the root to the ends.

4. Wait several minutes for the spray to set, and then remove the bobby pins.

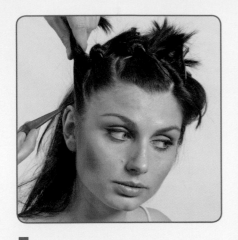

5.

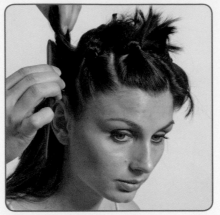

6.

5. Repeat this process all the way around the hairline to the nape of the neck.

6. Roll each section of hair into a rope, and gather the ends in a circle around the crown.

7. Secure each section with a bobby pin, leaving 1½-inches of hair loose at the ends.

8. For extra strength, tighten the twisted sections before securing them with bobby pins, and secure them as close to the root as you can. Take care when dividing the hair into sections since each section creates a visible part in the hair.

9. Insert pins through every rope of hair, toward the center of the head.

10. Gather the loose hair at the crown and divide it into two sections.

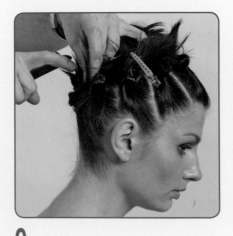

7.

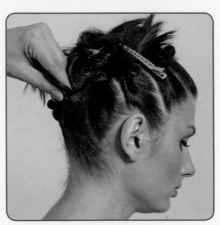

8.

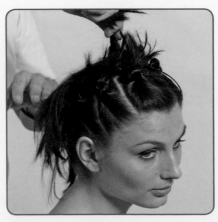

9.

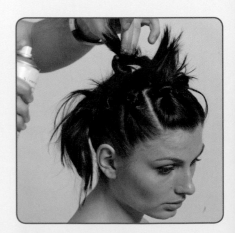

10.

11.

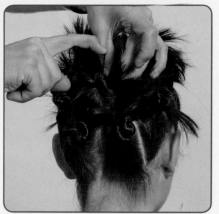

12

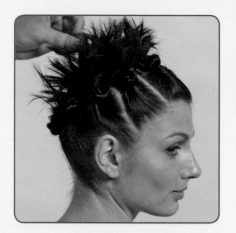

13

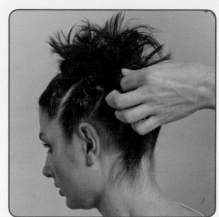

14

11. Twist each section into a rope and mist with holding spray.

12. Secure the ropes with bobby pins. Secure the hair with extra bobby pins and mist with holding spray.

13. Separate the ends of hair extending from each rope at the crown of the head.

14. Position the holding spray about 6 inches away and mist the hair.

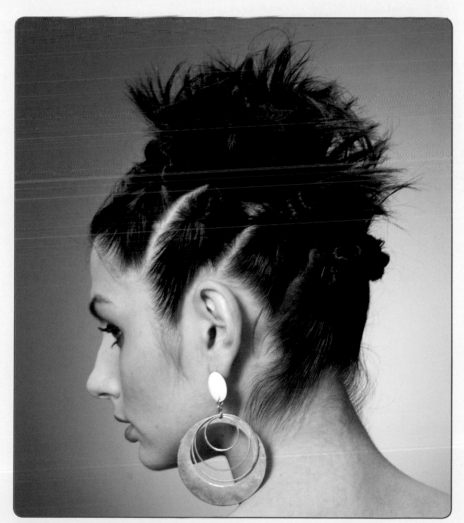

15

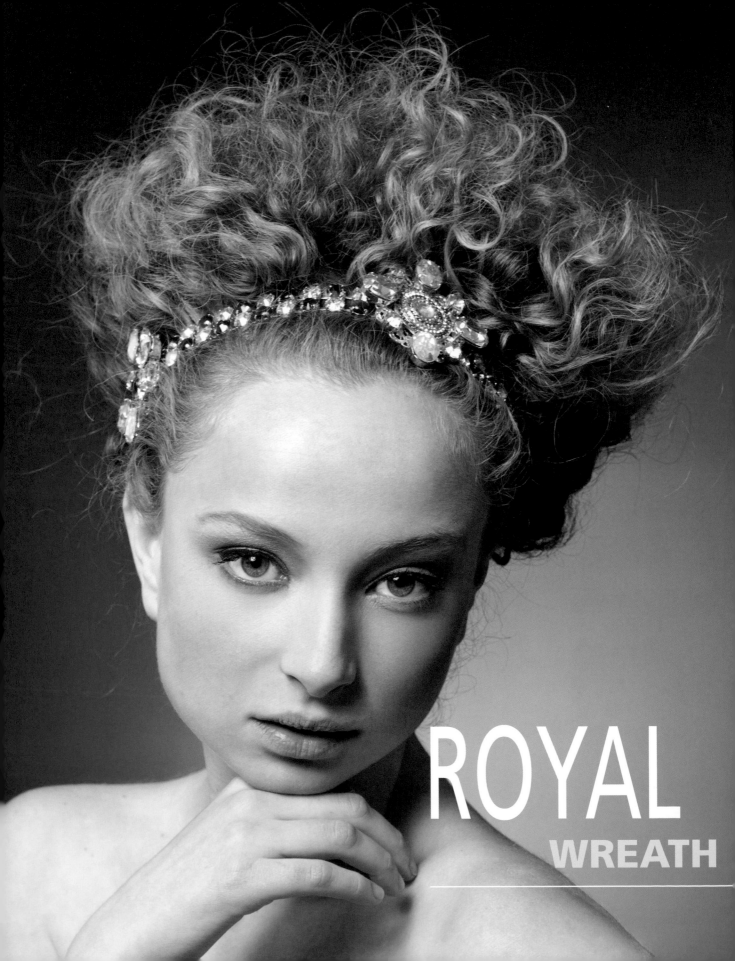

ROYAL
WREATH

29

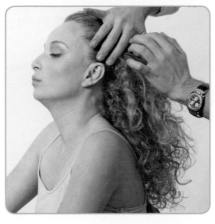

1. Wash and blow dry the hair. Apply molding wax by rubbing a bit of wax between your hands, then drawing your fingers through the curls.

2. Gather a section of hair on one side of the head, from just behind the ear to the brow.

3. Gently twist the gathered hair inward, and pull it toward the back of the head.

4. Tuck the ends of the hair under the twist, and secure at the top of the head with bobby pins.

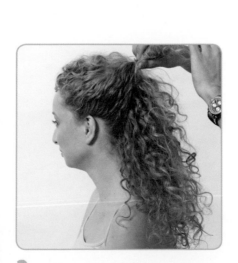

In this design, the brow and neck are exposed as the hair is swept up and away from the face. For greater elegance, add a jeweled hair band and decorated comb.

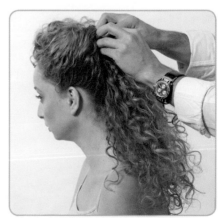

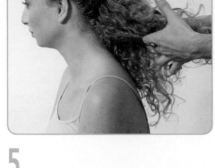

5

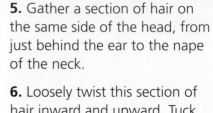
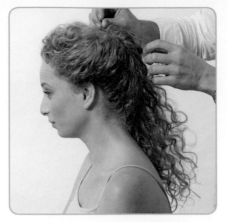

6

5. Gather a section of hair on the same side of the head, from just behind the ear to the nape of the neck.

6. Loosely twist this section of hair inward and upward. Tuck the ends under the hair, and secure the hair on top of the head near the place where the first section of hair was secured.

7. Repeat the same process on the other side of the head, starting with a section of hair from just behind the ear to the brow.

8. Twist the hair inward, and pull it toward the back of the head.

9. Check that the hair looks symmetrical at the front; then secure the twisted hair with bobby pins.

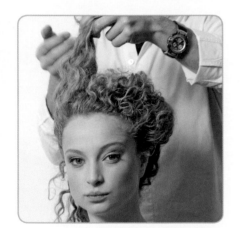

7

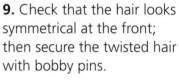

8

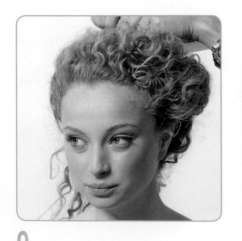

9

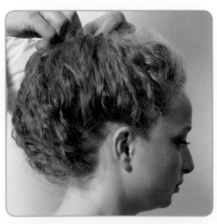

10

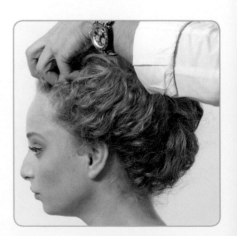

11

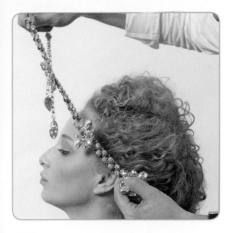
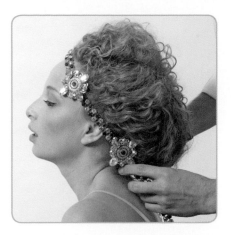
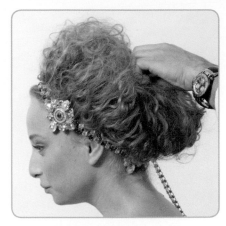

12 **13** **14**

10. Gather the remaining section of loose hair at the back of the head, and twist it upward and forward. Tuck in the ends, and secure the hair with bobby pins near the other sections of gathered hair.

11. Shape the hair with your fingers for an even, balanced look all around the head.

12. For a perfect finish, select a jeweled headband and position it around the head, just above the hairline.

13. Secure the headband at the nape of the neck.

14. Lift the ends of the headband upward and secure it to the hair with clips or bobby pins.

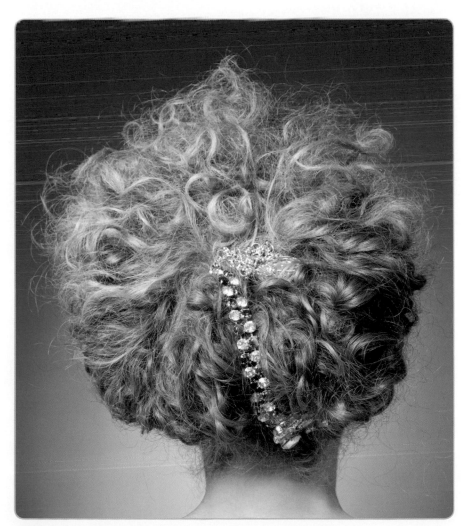

15

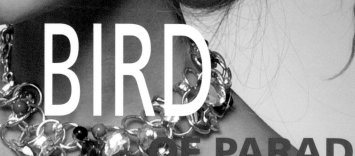

BIRD
OF PARADISE

30

With a combination of braided hair, crimped hair, and straight hair, this hairstyle is big and dramatic. It can be strikingly paired with a simple (or not so simple) black dress.

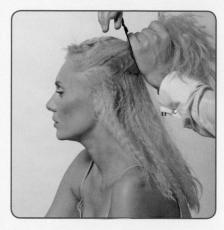

1

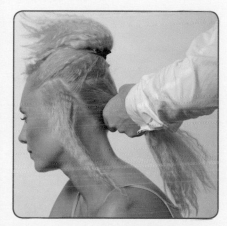

2

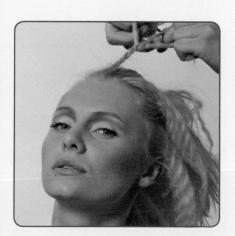

3

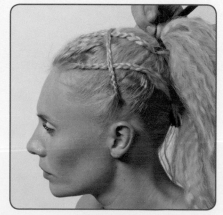

4

1. Wash the hair, apply styling mousse, and then blow dry. Crimp the hair with a crimping iron, starting at the roots and crimping all the away to the ends. For best results, hold the crimp iron for about 5 seconds each time. Make a horizontal part just above the ears and all the way around the back of the head. Leave the bangs loose, and gather the hair above the part at the bag of the head into a ponytail.

2. Make parts just behind both ears. Gather the hair between the parts into a low ponytail at the back of the head.

3. Gather the hair along the brow into small sections, and braid the hair backward. Secure each braid with a small elastic band at the end.

4. Draw the braids in diagonal directions over the top of the head, orienting all of them toward the ponytail. Secure the braids at the ends with bobby pins.

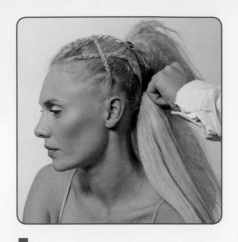

5

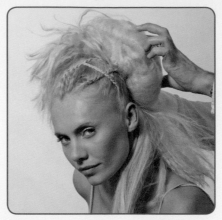

6

5. Select two long hair extensions that match the color of the hair. Affix one extension below the base of the ponytail.

6. Select a large sponge that matches the color of the hair, and shape it into a rectangle. Affix the sponge above the base of the ponytail.

7. Attach the other extension above the sponge.

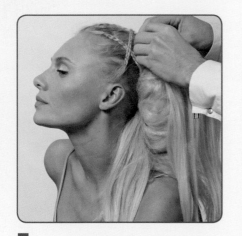

7

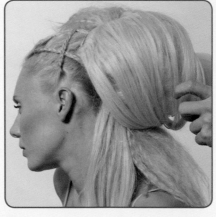

8

8. Cover the sponge with the hair extension and secure it with bobby pins. Mist the hair with holding spray.

9. Lift the hair extension affixed below the ponytail, and fold inward and upward. Twist the extension below the fold, and bring it up toward the sponge.

10. Secure the ends of the hair in front of the sponge, and backcomb the ends so that they flare up at the top of the head.

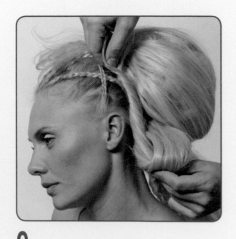

9

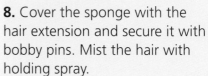

10

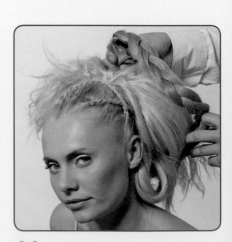

11

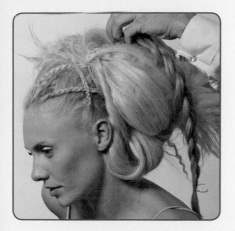

12

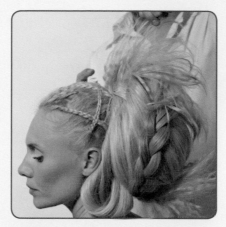

13

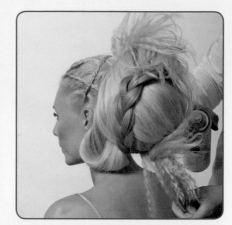

14

11. Select a hair extension that is a different shade from the color of the hair, and braid.

12. Secure the extension above the sponge and twist it around the sponge. Secure the bottom of the extension at the top of the sponge, close to the top of the extension.

13. Backcomb the loose ends of hair at the top of the head, and mist them with holding spray.

14. Mist the entire hairstyle to complete the look.

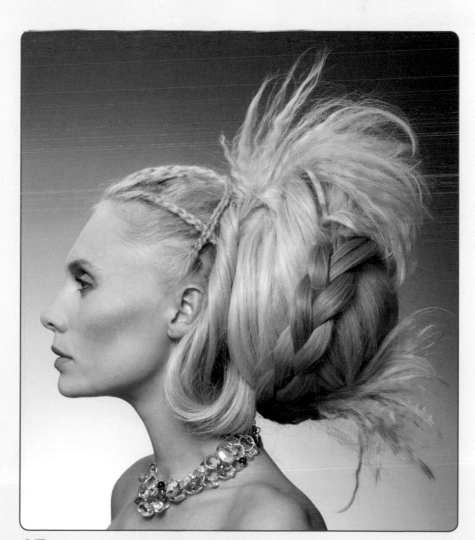

15

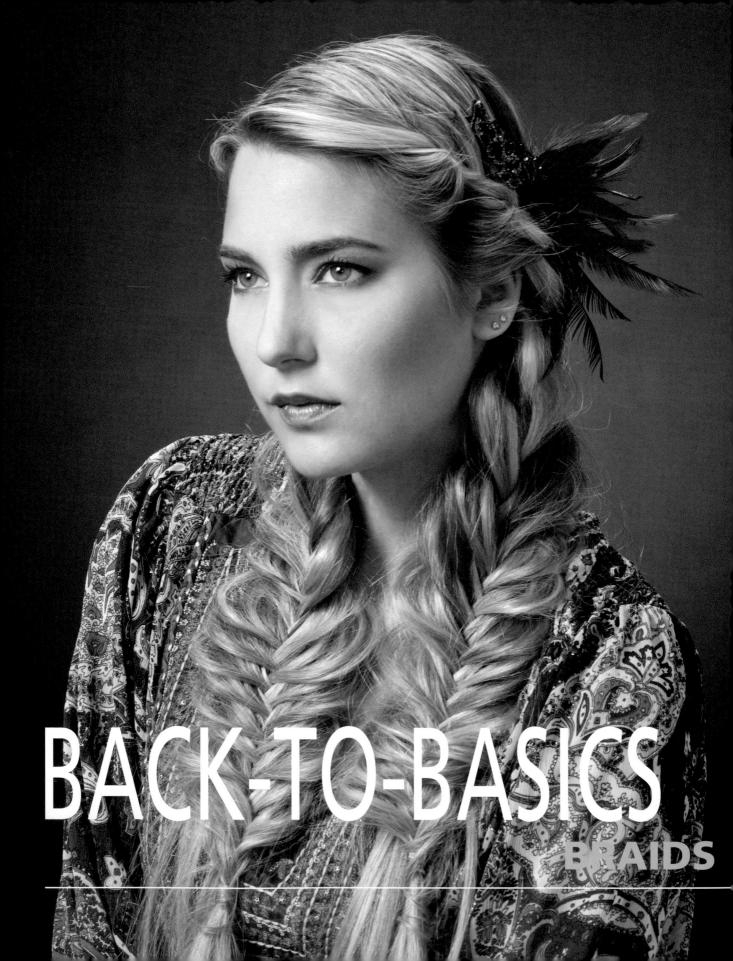

BACK-TO-BASICS
BRAIDS

31

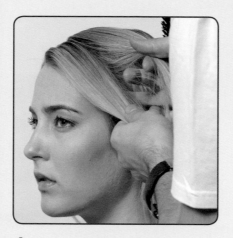

1

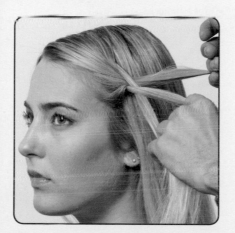

2

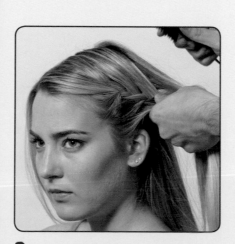

3

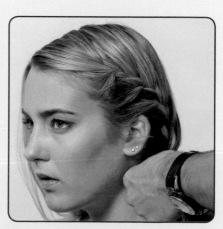

4

1. Wash and blow dry the hair. Make a deep side part and gather a section of hair above the part at the brow.

2. Divide this section of hair into three equal sections and start making a braid.

3. Continue braiding this section of hair along the side of the head, adding to each section of the braid as you proceed.

4. Comb the hair each time you add more hair to the braid, to maintain a unified look. Continue braiding the hair along the head and below the ear.

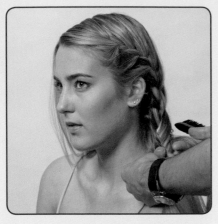

5

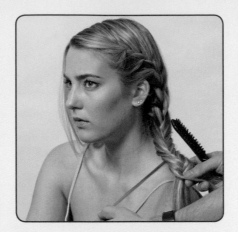

6

5. Divide the hair along the part into two sections. As you continue braiding the hair, integrate locks from the loose hair while making sure that all three sections of the braid are even.

6. Continue braiding the hair while integrating loose sections of hair. The braid should include all of the hair on one side of the part, from the brow to the crown.

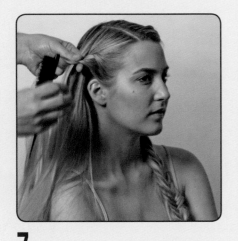

7

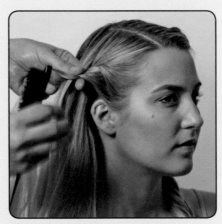

8

7. As you proceed with the bottom of the braid, draw thin locks of hair from each braided section and let them hang loose.

8. Secure the braid a few inches from the end with an elastic band. Begin braiding the hair on the other side of the head, starting with the hair at the brow.

9. Repeat the entire process on the other side of the head.

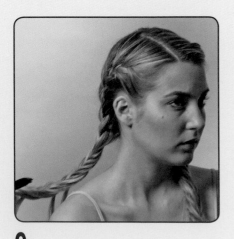

9

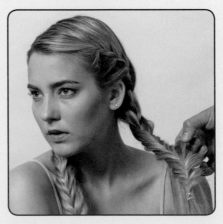

10

10. Secure the second braid near the end with an elastic band. Return to the first braid and gently tug at several locks from the braid, to loosen them, while holding the end of the braid. Do not pull the locks out of the braid.

11. Proceed this way all the way up to the roots of the braid.

12. Backcomb the loose ends of the braid with your fingers.

13. Repeat this process on the second braid.

14. Proceed all the way up to the roots of the braid.

15. Use bobby pins to secure the braided hair to the head, if necessary.

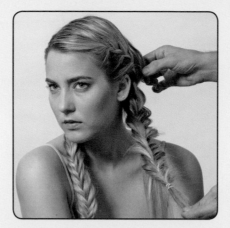

11

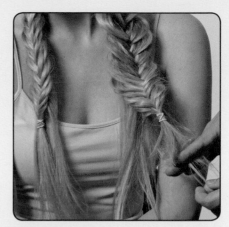

12

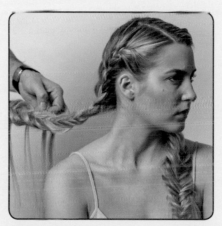

13

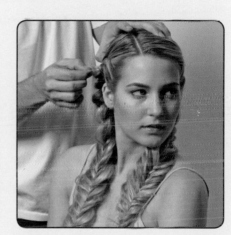

14

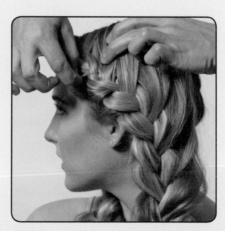

15

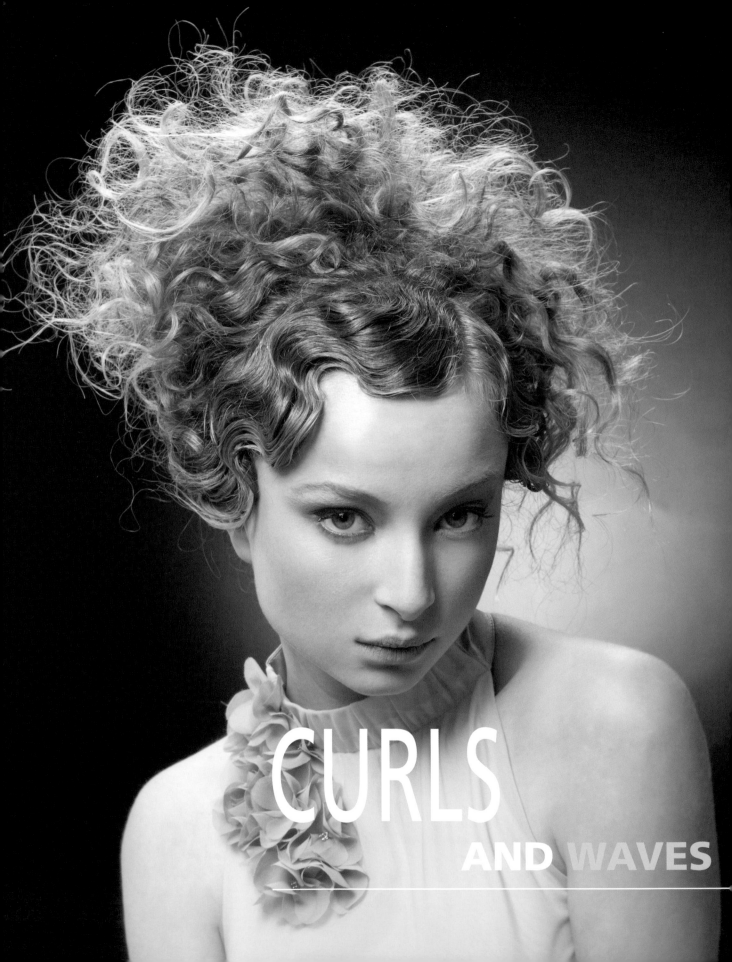

CURLS
AND WAVES

32

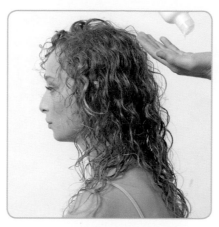

1. Wash and towel dry the hair. Apply moisturizing cream with your hands.

2. Apply liquid gel to the hair for maximum maintenance of natural curls.

3. Apply the gel to your hands first; then scrunch the hair to distribute the gel evenly throughout the hair.

4. To tighten the curls, grasp separate locks of hair and twist them.

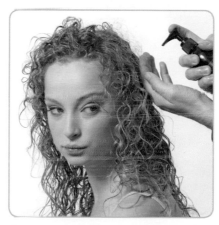

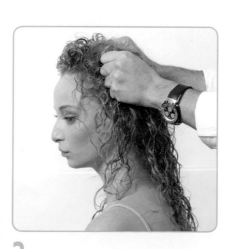

This hairstyle makes a statement by maximizing curly hair. The front of the hairstyle is carefully sculpted and styled, while the back is curly and carefree.

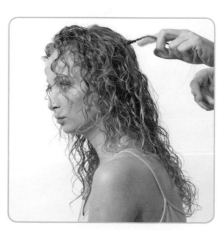

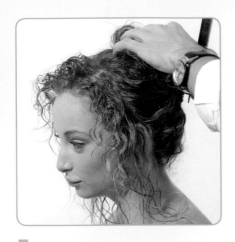

5

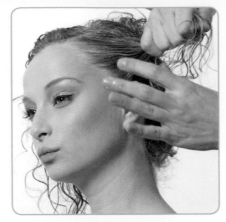

6

5. Divide the hair into front and back sections. The front section should be about 2½-inches wide, from the brow to the top of the head. Leave the front section loose. Gather the back section at the back of the head and secure with a clip.

6. Apply liquid gel to the loose hair at the front, and draw the hair to one side of the head backward.

7. Make a deep side part in the loose hair at the other side of the front, and draw the hair above the part across the brow, to the other side of the head. Secure the hair with a clip.

8. Shape the hair on the other side of the part to create a small wave, and secure it with a clip.

9. Repeat the process as you work your way along the brow and down the side of the face, creating waves and securing each wave with a clip.

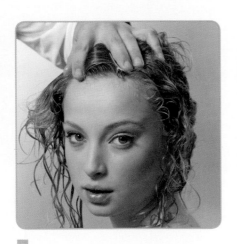

7

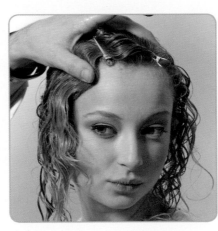

8

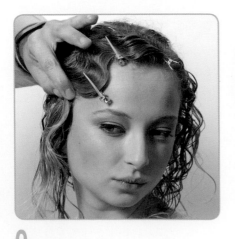

9

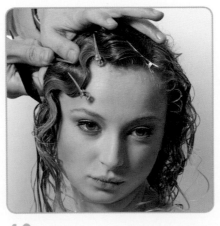

10

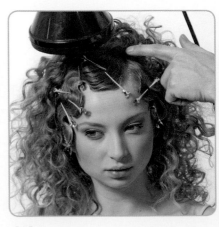

11

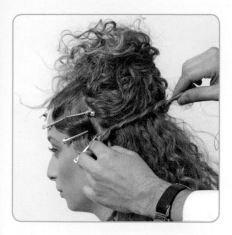

12

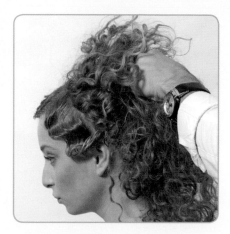

13

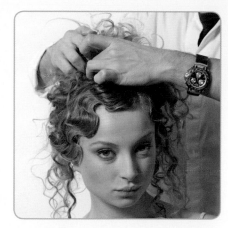

14

10. Sculpt the waves as desired, and secure them with clips.

11. Dry the hair with a diffuser to set the waves at the front of the head. Release the hair at the back of the head.

12. Move to the back section of hair. Select a lock of hair above one ear and twist it tightly from the roots to the ends. Secure the twisted hair with bobby pins below the crown.

13. Gather the hair in the back section.

14. Secure the hair in random groups with small elastic bands to create a free, natural look. To complete the look, loosen several long strands along the back and sides.

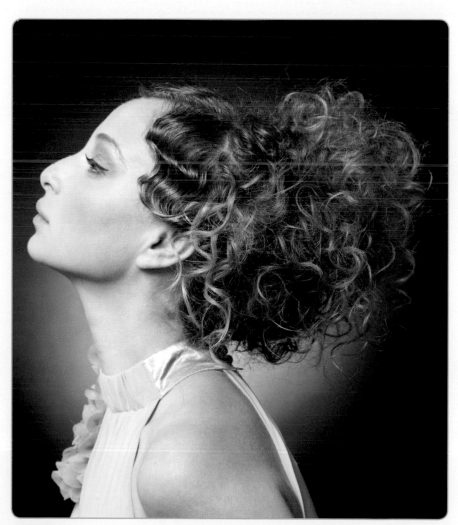

15

SWIRLING
SIREN

33

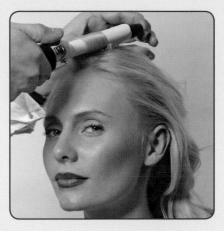

1

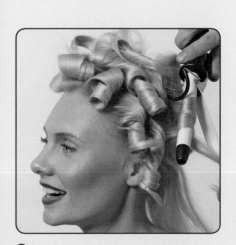

2

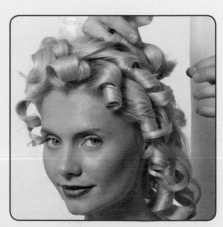

3

4

1. Wash and blow dry the hair. Separate a small section of hair at the crown and curl with a small curling iron.

2. Continue curling the hair, section by section, starting at the top of the head and moving downward along the brow.

3. Continue curling the hair to the nape of the neck on one side; then move to the other side and curl all of the hair. Mist with holding spray as you go.

4. Loosen one of the curls at the back of the head with your fingers, and comb it gently.

This swirled design features dozens of curled locks, styled randomly at the back of the hair. A romantic salute to Hollywood's most glorious screen sirens.

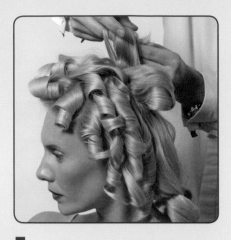

5

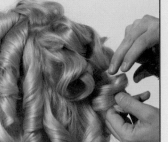
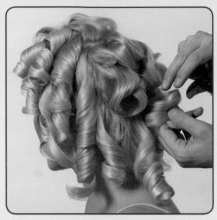

6

5. Roll the curl around your fingers, work it into a wavelike shape, and secure the ends to the head with bobby pins.

6. Repeat this process with the rest of the curls at the back of the head.

7. If necessary, backcomb the hair at the roots for extra volume, but take care not to damage the curls as you comb.

8. Move to the front of the head and loosen a curl near the brow. Draw the curl backward and secure the ends to the head with bobby pins.

9. Repeat this process with the rest of the curls at the front of the head. Secure these waves in a manner that maintains volume and adds height at the front.

10. Repeat this process at the sides of the head.

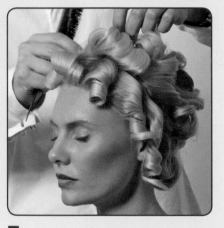

7

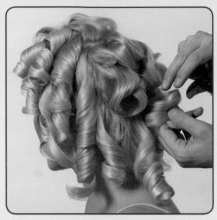

8

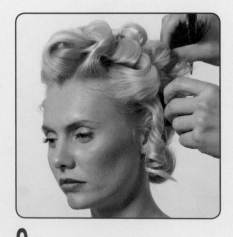

9

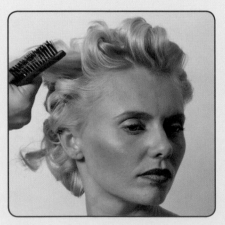

10

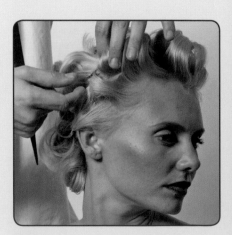

11

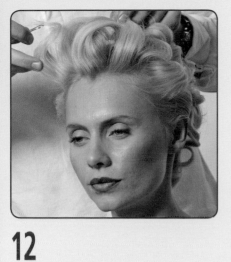

12

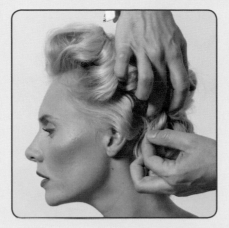

13

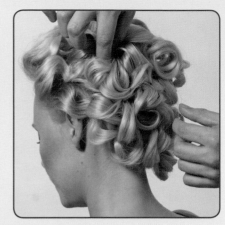

14

11. Continue the process until all of the curls are secured.

12. Use clips to style the hair as desired; then mist the hair with holding spray.

13. Arrange the bangs for maximum height at the front. Add bobby pins as needed for longstanding hold.

14. Make final adjustments; then mist the hair with holding spray.

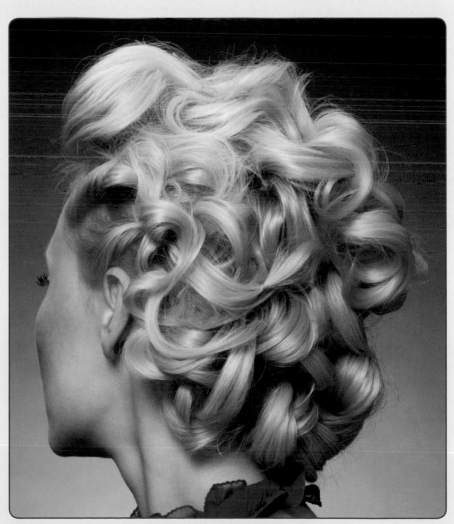

15

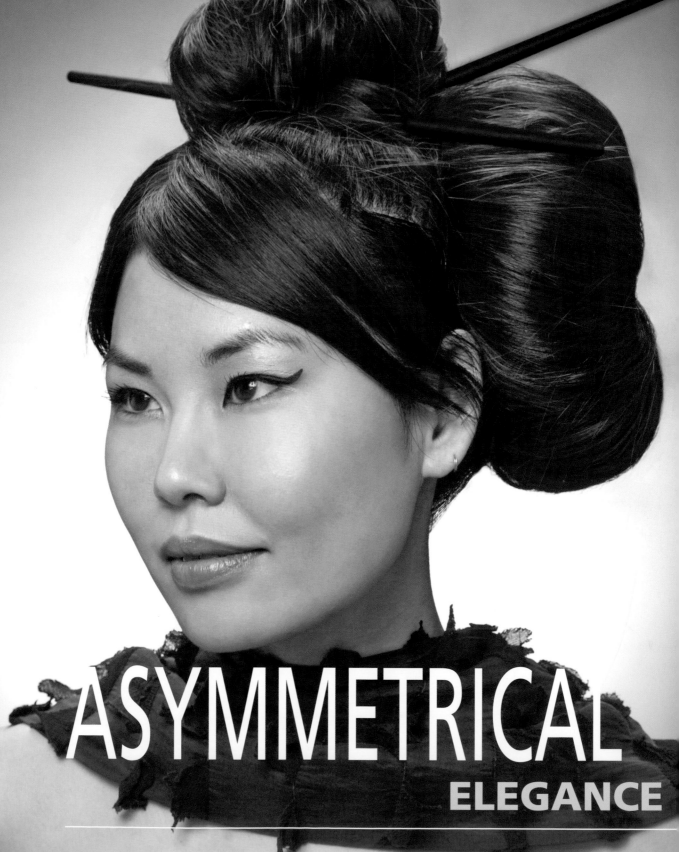

ASYMMETRICAL
ELEGANCE

34

With two oversized buns and two thick wooden accessories, this hairstyle is a modern take on a traditional design.

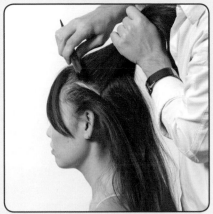

1

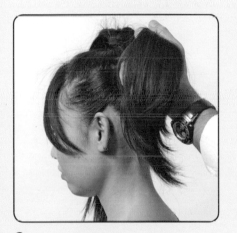

2

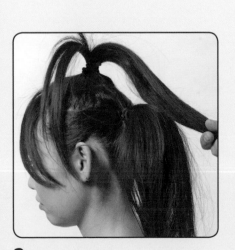

3

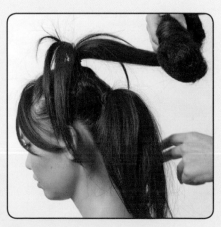

4

1. Wash and blow dry the hair. Gather a section of hair at the front of the head, leaving the hair at the bangs and just above the ears loose. Secure the hair in a ponytail.

2. Brush back the hair from just above the ears, and gather it, along with the rest of the hair at the back of the head, below the first ponytail.

3. Separate the hair in the top ponytail into a top and bottom section. The bottom sections should be about three times thicker than the top section.

4. Select a small sponge that matches the color of the hair, and place it on the ends of the larger section of hair in the top ponytail.

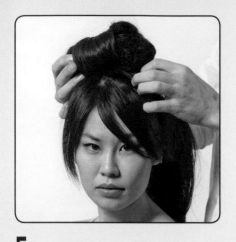

5

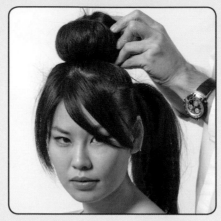

6

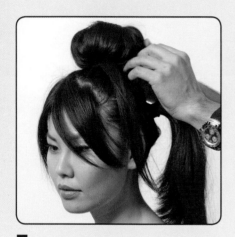

7

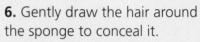

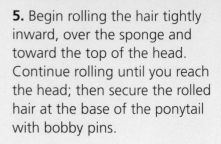

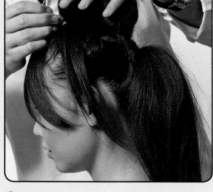

8

5. Begin rolling the hair tightly inward, over the sponge and toward the top of the head. Continue rolling until you reach the head; then secure the rolled hair at the base of the ponytail with bobby pins.

6. Gently draw the hair around the sponge to conceal it.

7. Make sure the hair is rolled tightly around the sponge, and twist it as you roll to form a coil. Secure the hair at the top of the head, near the base of the ponytail.

8. Insert bobby pins all around the base of the rolled hair to affix it in place and maintain the shape.

9. Select another small sponge that matches the color of the hair. Place the sponge on the ends of the bottom ponytail and roll the hair tightly inward, over the sponge and toward the side of the head.

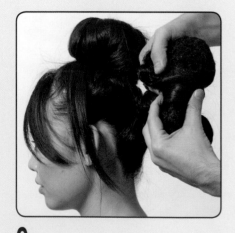

9

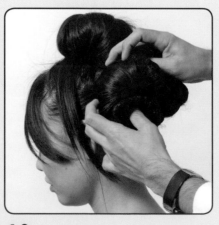

10

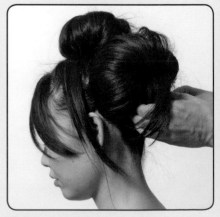

11

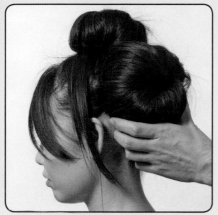 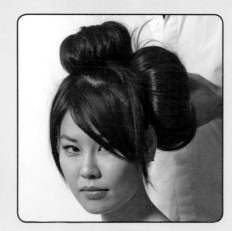 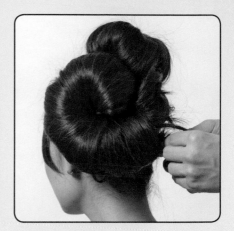

12 **13** **14**

10. Make sure the hair is rolled tightly around the sponge, and twist it as you roll to form a coil.

11. Secure the coiled hair at the side of the head, just below the base of the ponytail.

12. Insert bobby pins all around the rolled hair to secure it in place.

13. Secure loose ends to the coils with bobby pins. Smooth the bangs on either side of the face so that they frame it.

14. Mist the hair with holding spray. Insert two thick black sticks between the two coils to complete the hairstyle.

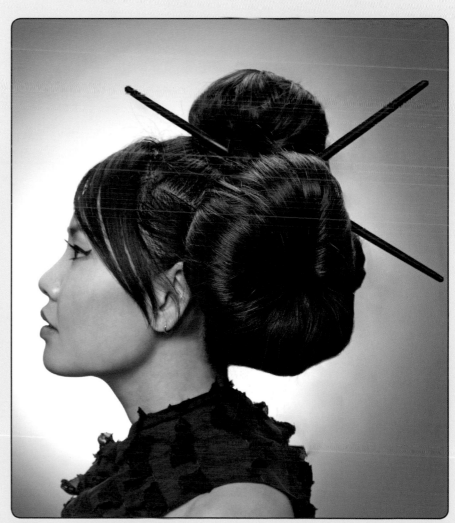

15

ROMANTIC
SIDE SWEEP

35

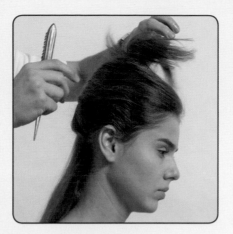

1

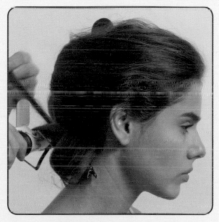

3

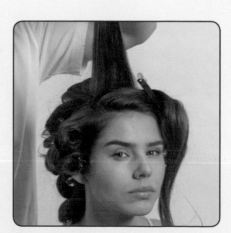

2

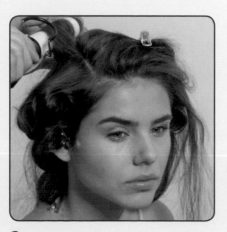

4

1. Wash and blow dry the hair.

2. Curl the hair with a medium curling iron, starting from the nape of the neck and moving up toward the brow.

3. Hold each lock in the curling iron for about 10 seconds and mist each one with holding spray.

4. Secure each curled lock to the head with bobby pins until set.

This soft style features a side part and several gentle curls. A romantic hairstyle inspired by a 1940s coiffure, it's perfect for any special occasion.

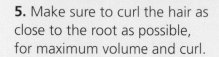

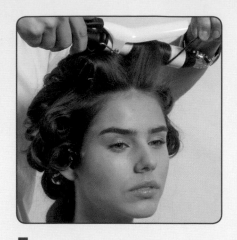

5

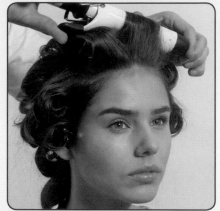

6

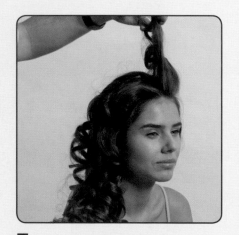

7

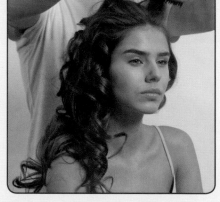

8

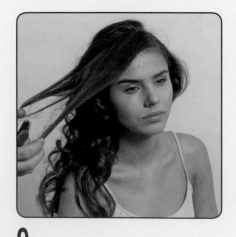

9

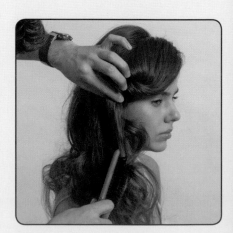

10

11

5. Make sure to curl the hair as close to the root as possible, for maximum volume and curl.

6. Curl the bangs so that curls are positioned away from the face.

7. Once the curls have had a chance to set, remove the bobby pins and gently the loosen curls with your fingers. Mist the loose hair with holding spray.

8. Comb the bangs to one side.

9. Divide the bangs into two sections and twist the sections together.

10. Draw the twisted bangs gently toward the back of the head, and secure them at the crown.

11. Gently comb the loose hair.

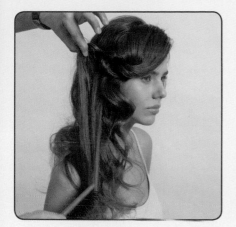

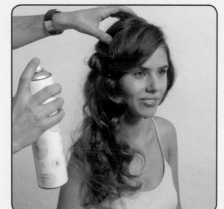

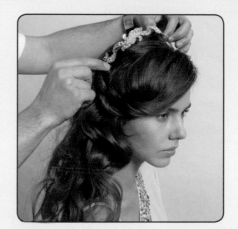

12

13

14

12. Combing over the curled hair will create a look reminiscent of the 1940s.

13. Position the holding spray about 6 inches away and mist the hair.

14. Add a tiara to complete the look.

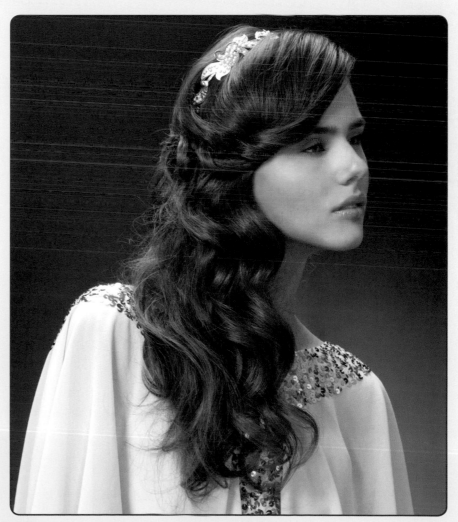

15

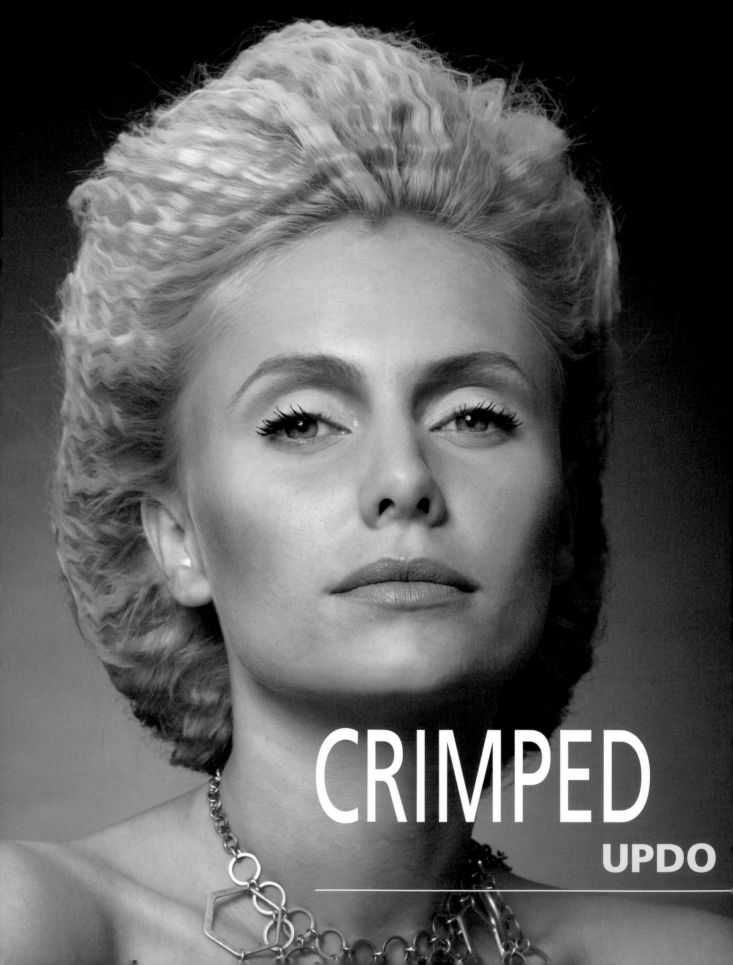

CRIMPED

UPDO

36

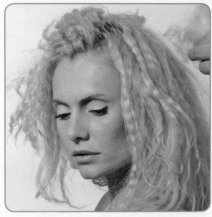

1

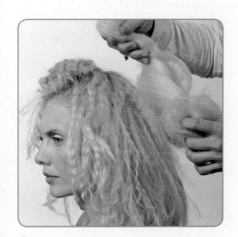

2

1. Wash the hair, apply styling mousse, and then blow dry. Crimp the hair with a crimping iron, starting at the roots and crimping all the away to the ends. For best results, hold the crimp iron for about 5 seconds each time.

2. Select a long, wide sponge that matches the color of the hair.

3. Shape the sponge into a ring, and arrange it on the head in the form of a crown.

4. Secure the sponge firmly with bobby pins.

This hairstyle combines crimped locks with a large hair sponge to create a dramatic, textured look that is funky and elegant at the same time.

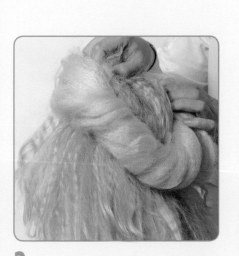

3

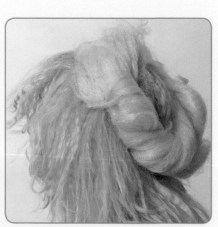

4

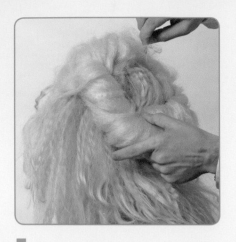

5

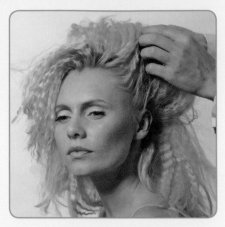

6

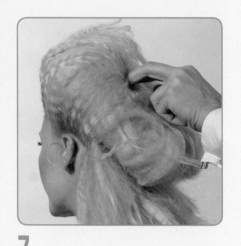

7

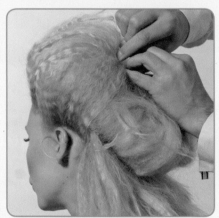

8

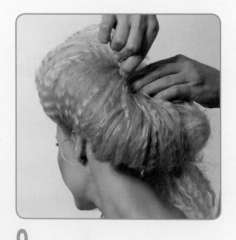

9

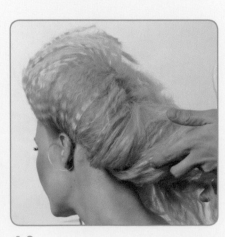

10

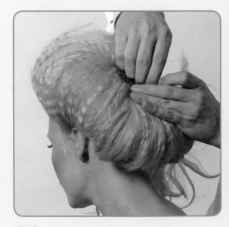

11

5. Make sure the sponge is secure, as it is the base of this hairstyle.

6. Begin drawing the loose hair upward to cover the sponge. Start at the front of head, above the ear, and draw the hair upward and over the sponge.

7. Secure the hair in the center of the head with bobby pins.

8. Continue to work your way around the ring, drawing the hair upward and toward the center of the head. Use your fingers, rather than a comb, to draw the hair upward to avoid damaging the crimp.

9. Continue this process all around the hairline.

10. Draw up the hair at the nape of the neck as well. Mist the hair with holding spray after it is secured.

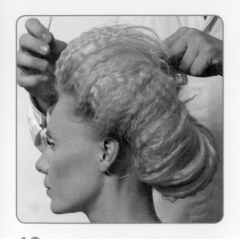

12

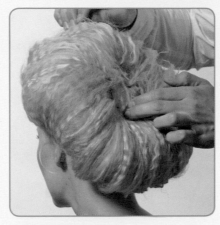

13

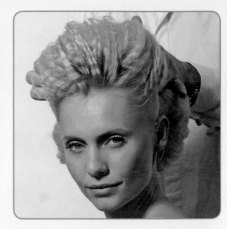

14

11. Spread out the hair over the sponge so that the sponge is completely concealed.

12. Repeat this process until all the hair has been secured.

13. Add bobby pins as required to secure the hairstyle.

14. Shape the hair with your fingers as desired. Mist it with holding spray to secure.

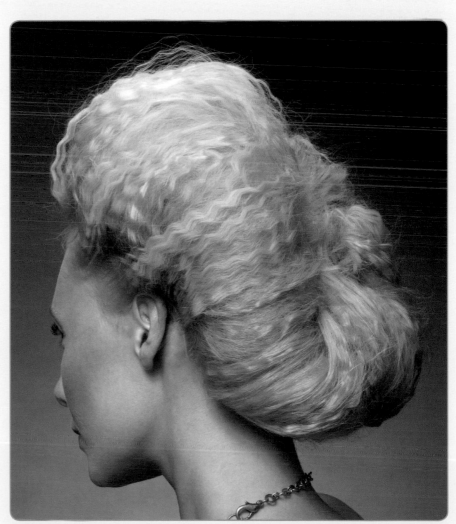

15

SCHOOLGIRL
ELEGANCE

37

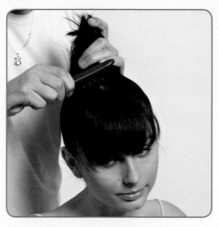

1

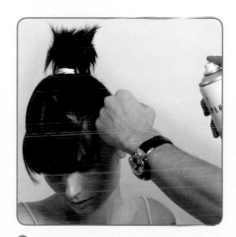

2

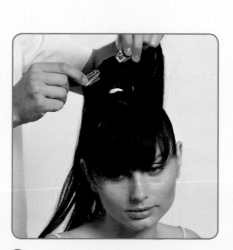

3

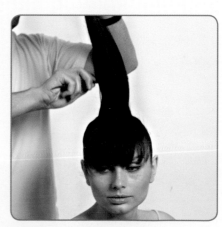

4

1. Wash and blow dry the hair. Brush the bangs forward and gather the rest of the hair in a high ponytail.

2. Position the holding spray about 6 inches away, and mist the hair while combing it through.

3. Select a hair extension that matches the color of the hair. Attach the extension to the base of the ponytail with bobby pins.

4. Brush the hair and hair extension together to integrate them. Mist the hair lightly with holding spray.

This hairstyle combines the girlish charm of bangs with the elegance of a high updo. It highlights the eyes, which are framed by the bangs, and shows off a beautifully bare neck.

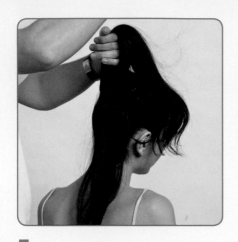

5

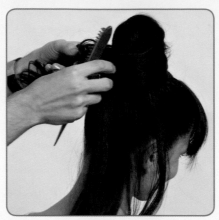

6

5. Separate a lock from the bottom of the gathered hair. Backcomb the rest of the hair in the ponytail.

6. Twist the ponytail around its base to form a thick bun.

7. Use a clip to secure the twisted ponytail in place.

8. Secure the twisted hair with bobby pins.

9. Divide the separated lock into two sections.

10. Twist the sections together to form a rope.

11. Continue twisting the sections all the way to the end.

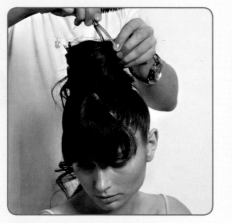

7

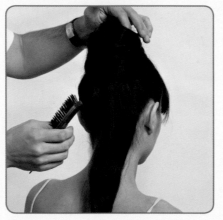

8

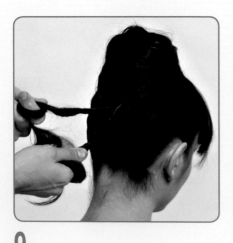

9

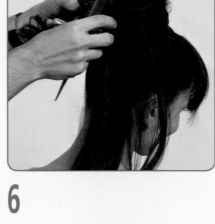

10

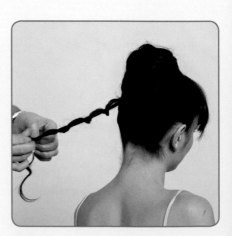

11

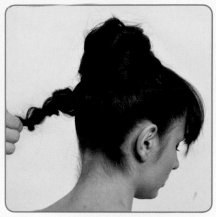

12

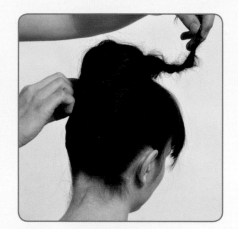

13

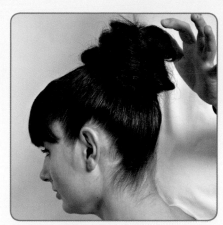

14

12. Push the twisted section of hair toward the root to create a natural texture.

13. Wrap this section of hair around the base of the bun.

14. Secure the twisted section of hair with bobby pins. Position the holding spray about 6 inches away and mist the hair.

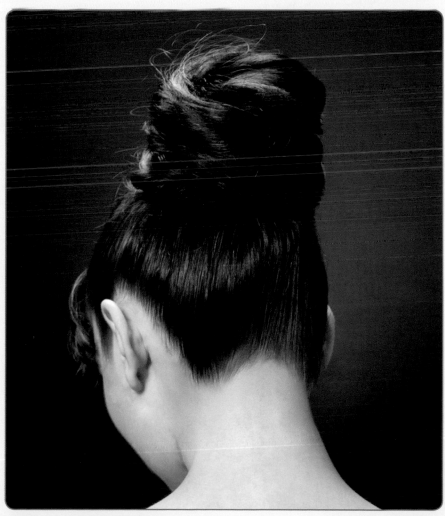

15

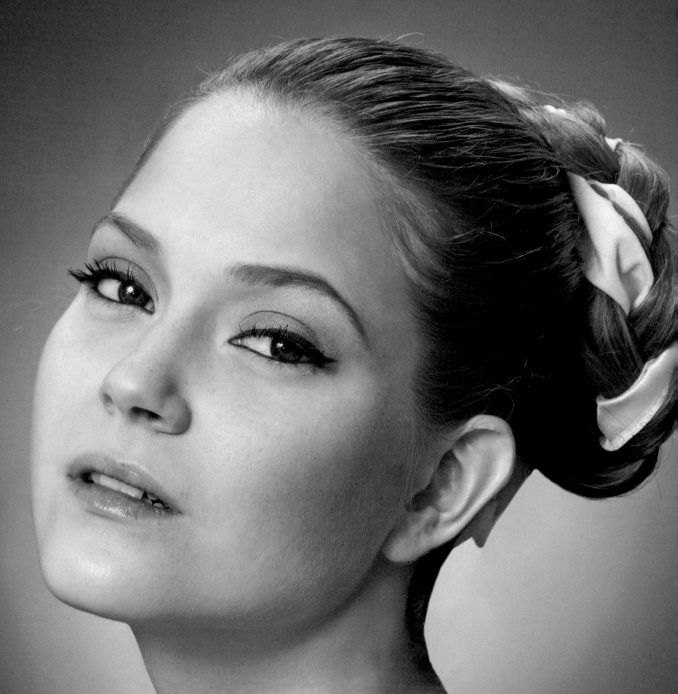

WRAPPED

WITH A RIBBON

38

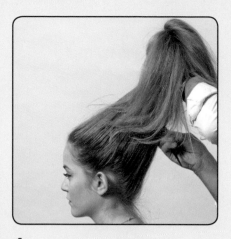

1 Wash and blow dry the hair. Hold the hair at the ends and comb it in an upward motion.

2. Gather the hair in a high ponytail at the back of the head.

3. Secure the ponytail hair with an elastic band.

1

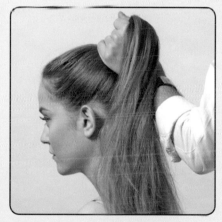

2

With its thick ivory ribbon, this pretty hairstyle looks like a present just waiting to be opened. Replace the ribbon to suit your mood, outfit, and occasion.

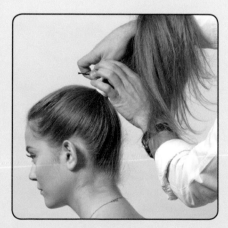

3

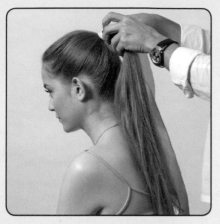

4

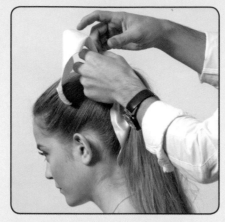

5

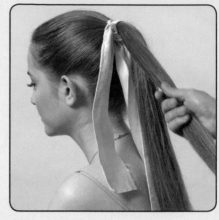

6

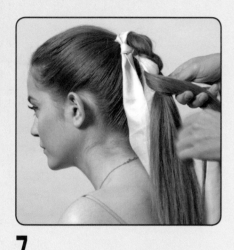

7

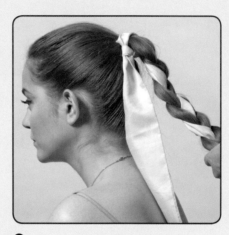

8

4. Tie a 20-inch ribbon securely around the base of the ponytail. Choose a ribbon that matches or contrasts with your outfit.

5. When tying the ribbon, make sure that one end is about twice as long as the other.

6. Divide the hair into three even sections.

7. Join the ribbon to one of the sections, and begin braiding the hair.

8. Braid the hair all the way to the ends. Make sure the ribbon remains smooth as you braid.

9. Secure the braid at the end with an elastic band.

10. Fold the braid upward from the base.

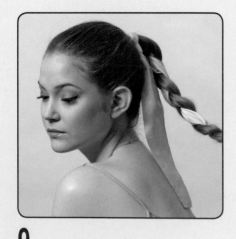

9

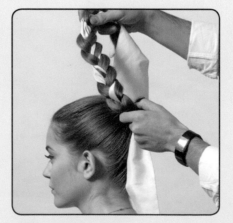

10

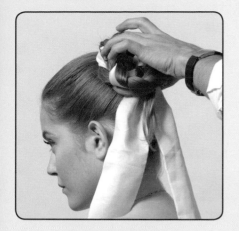

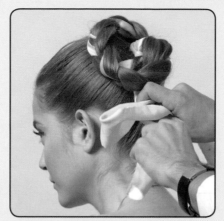

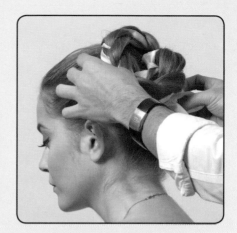

11

12

11. Wrap the braid over the top of the base and bring it around to the other side, then toward the bottom of the base, to make a braided bun. Secure the bun with bobby pins.

12. Tie the ends of ribbon together in a bow to complete the look.

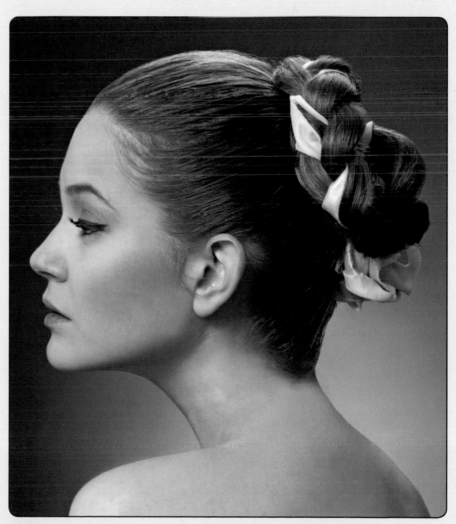

13

SWEPT
AWAY

39

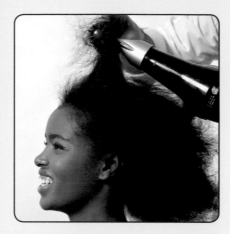

1

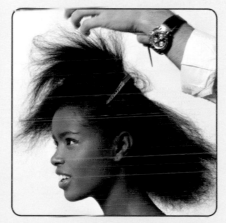

2

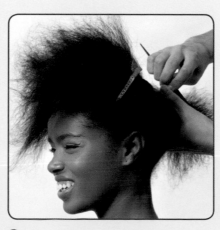

3

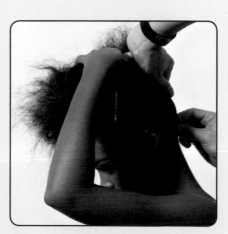

4

1. Wash and blow dry the hair straight.

2. Make a part extending from the back of each ear around the back of the head, and brush the hair above the part upward and forward. Secure it with a clip.

3. Brush the hair at the back of the head behind the right ear backwards towards the middle of the head.

4. Fold over the ends and secure the hair with bobby pins.

This hairstyle is dramatic and bold. Highlighted with a couple of colorful hair bands and a pair of striking earrings, it is vivacious and exciting.

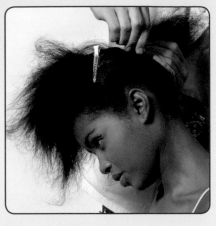

5

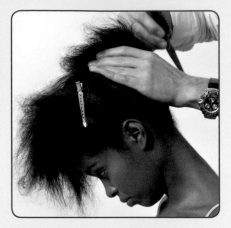

6

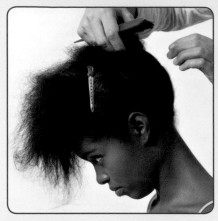

7

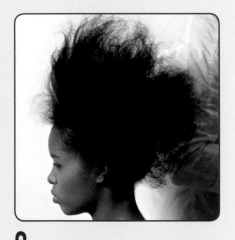

8

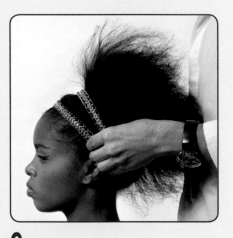

9

5. Brush the hair behind the left ear backwards and towards the middle of the head. Fold over the ends and mist the holding spray to secure.

6. Backcomb the hair ends at the back of the head to add volume.

7. Twist the hair ends upward to create a banana-shape that covers the line of bobby pins at the back, and secure it at the crown.

8. Release the hair at the front of the head from the clip, and backcomb to create volume.

9. Place a headband at the front of the head. Place a second, different but complementary, headband at the front of the head. The headbands highlight the contrast between the two different elements of the hairstyle.

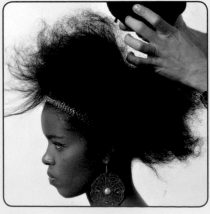

10

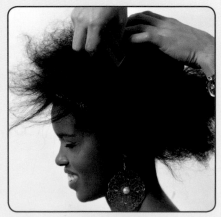

11

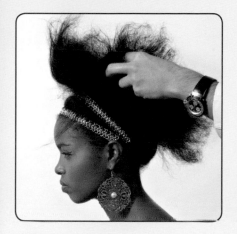

12

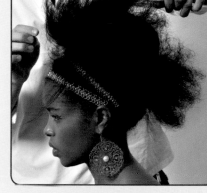

13

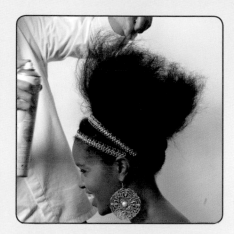

14

10. Select a sponge that matches the color of the hair, and shape it into a ball.

11. Secure the sponge at the crown of the head with bobby pins.

12. Arrange the natural hair around sponge to conceal it.

13. Secure several locks to the sponge with bobby pins.

14. To complete the look, mist the hair with holding spray and use your fingers to shape the ends of the standing hair.

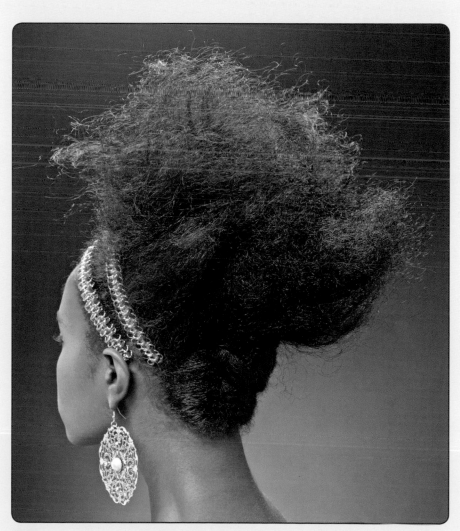

15

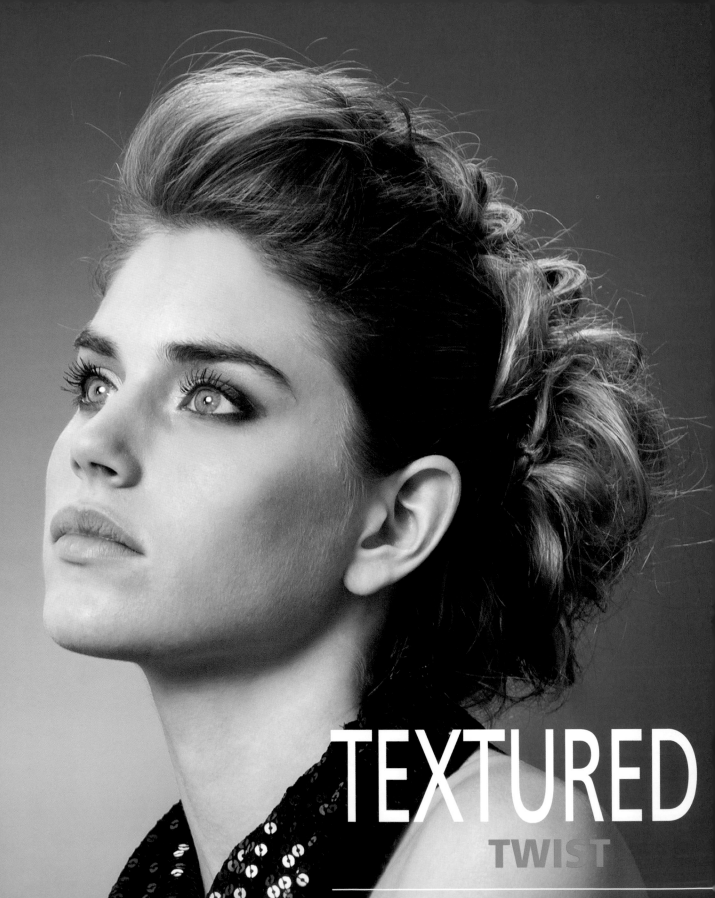

TEXTURED
TWIST

40

This playful design features several twisted locks that are swept up and away, exposing a bare neck and creating a soft, clean frame around the face. Enhance the look with a delicate pin.

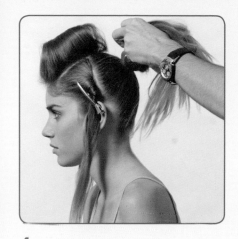

1

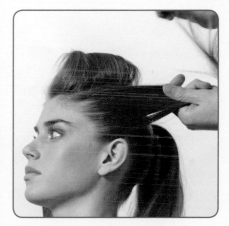

2

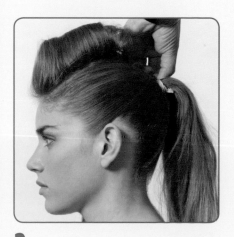

3

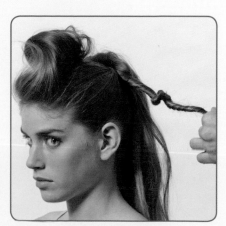

4

1. Wash and blow dry the hair. Make a part that extends from the top of each ear over the crown, and gather the hair below the part into a ponytail.

2. Divide the hair above the part into three sections, and brush the hair at the sides toward the ponytail at the back. Hold the hair at the middle of the brow in a clip.

3. Mist the hair at the sides with holding spray; then integrate it with the ponytail at the back of the head.

4. Grasp a lock of hair from the ponytail and twist it around itself.

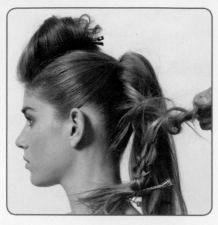

5

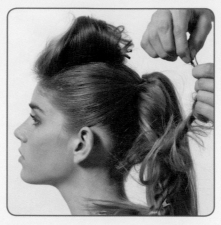

6

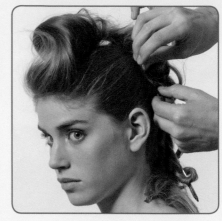

7

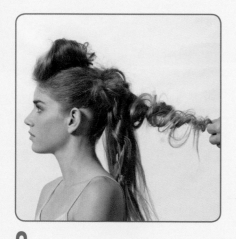

8

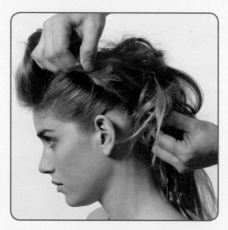

9

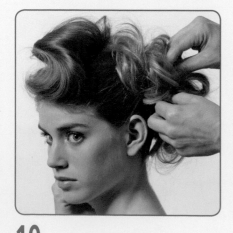

10

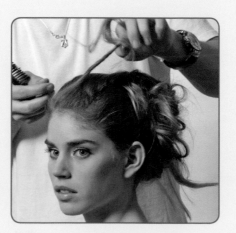

11

5. Hold the twisted lock at the ends and backcomb it loosely with your fingers.

6. Wrap the twisted ends around an open clip several times; then let the clip close to hold the twisted hair in place. Grasp another lock of hair from the ponytail and repeat the process.

7. Secure the twisted lock of hair near the base of the ponytail.

8. Continue twisting, backcombing, and roll the hair in the ponytail, section by section.

9. Secure the ends of each twisted lock of hair at the base of the ponytail with clips.

10. Repeat this process with the entire ponytail.

11. Release the hair at the middle of the brow from the clip and brush it backward.

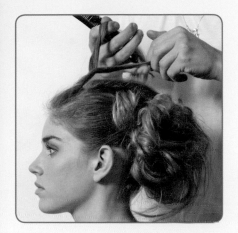

12

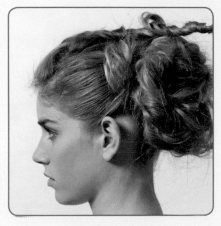

13

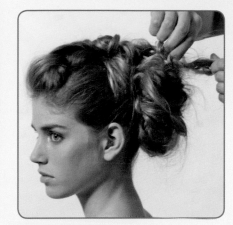

14

12. Divide this hair into two sections, and twist them together while drawing them backward.

13. Hold the ends of the twisted hair, and gently backcomb the hair with your fingers to loosen the twist.

14. Secure this twisted lock at the top of the ponytail. For a casual finish, gently pull at several locks in the bun. Mist the hair with holding spray to secure.

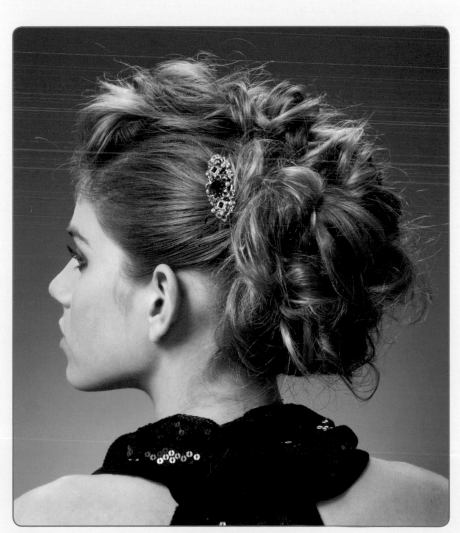

15

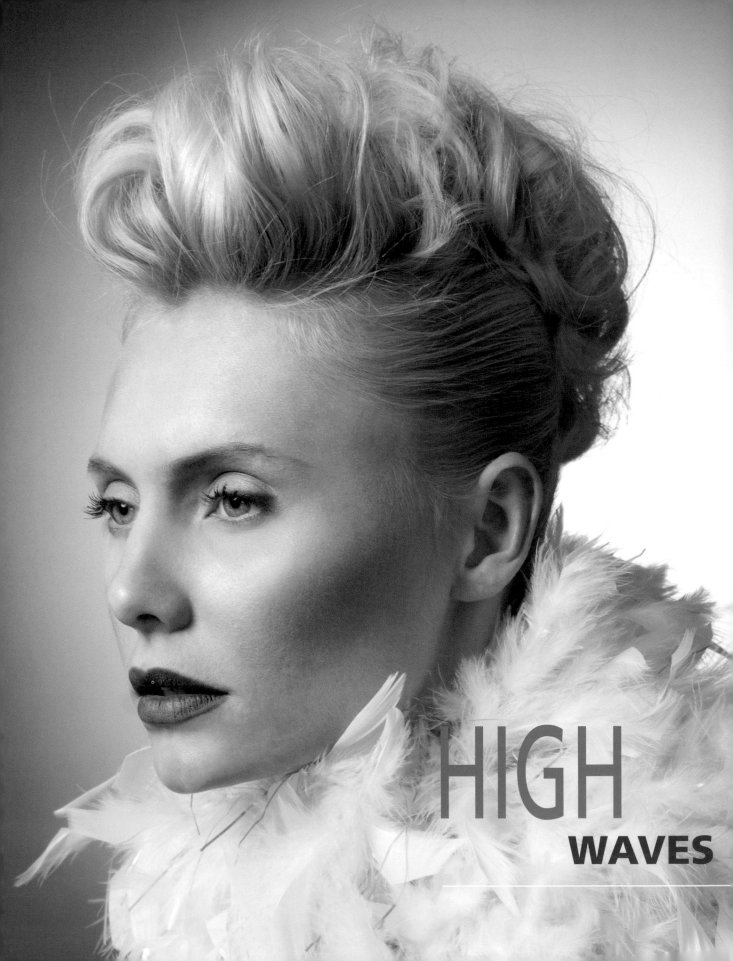

HIGH
WAVES

41

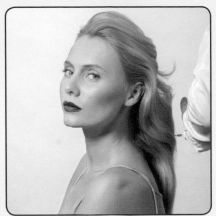

1

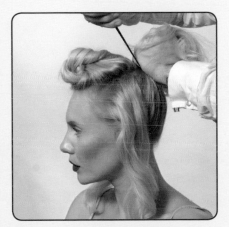

2

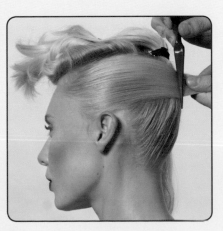

3

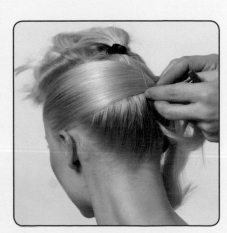

4

1. Wash and blow dry the hair wavy.

2. Divide the hair into three sections extending from the brow to the nape of the neck. Gather the hair at the back of the head into a high ponytail.

3. Mist the hair above one ear with holding spray, and comb it backward.

4. Make sure the hair is smooth and tight against the head; then secure it with a hairpin below the ponytail.

This hairstyle is striking yet soft. The smooth sides contrast with a wavy top, creating a multifaceted and dramatic design.

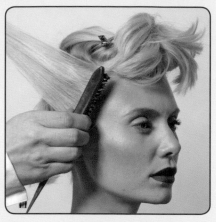

5

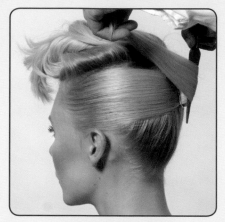

6

5. Repeat this process on the opposite side of the head.

6. Join the two sections of hair at the back of the head and comb upward.

7. Twist the hair into a vertical roll, and secure it by inserting a hairpin vertically, from the top to the bottom of the roll.

8. Wrap the hair at the crown of the head around the base of the ponytail.

9. Divide the loose hair at the top of the head into ½-inch wide sections, and backcomb each section.

10. Fold the sections of hair backward, and secure the ends to the roots with bobby pins.

11. Mist the hair with holding spray while styling the folded sections of hair.

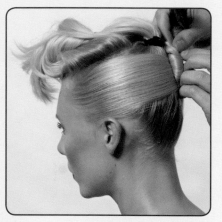

7

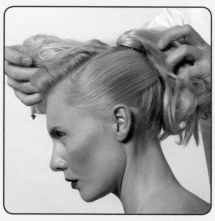

8

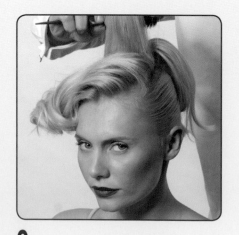

9

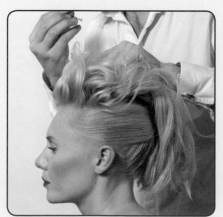

10

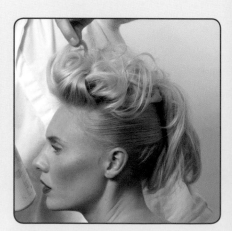

11

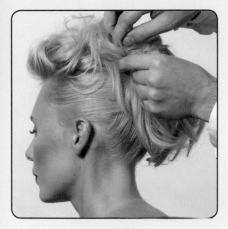

12

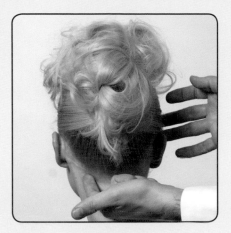

13

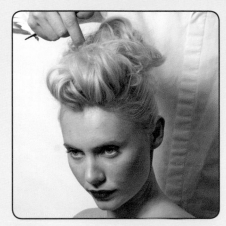

14

12. Continue styling and folding the hair, securing loose pieces of hair with bobby pins all the way to the ponytail.

13. Style the hair in the ponytail upward, in a similar fashion, to reach the hair at the top, and secure it with bobby pins.

14. Style the hair with your fingers to create a casual look at the top that contrasts with the neatness at the sides and back. Mist the hair with holding spray.

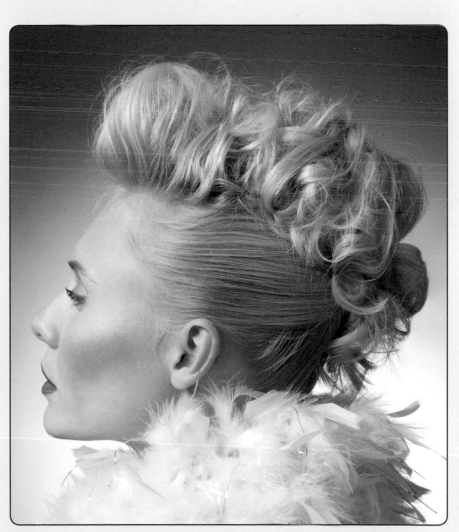

15

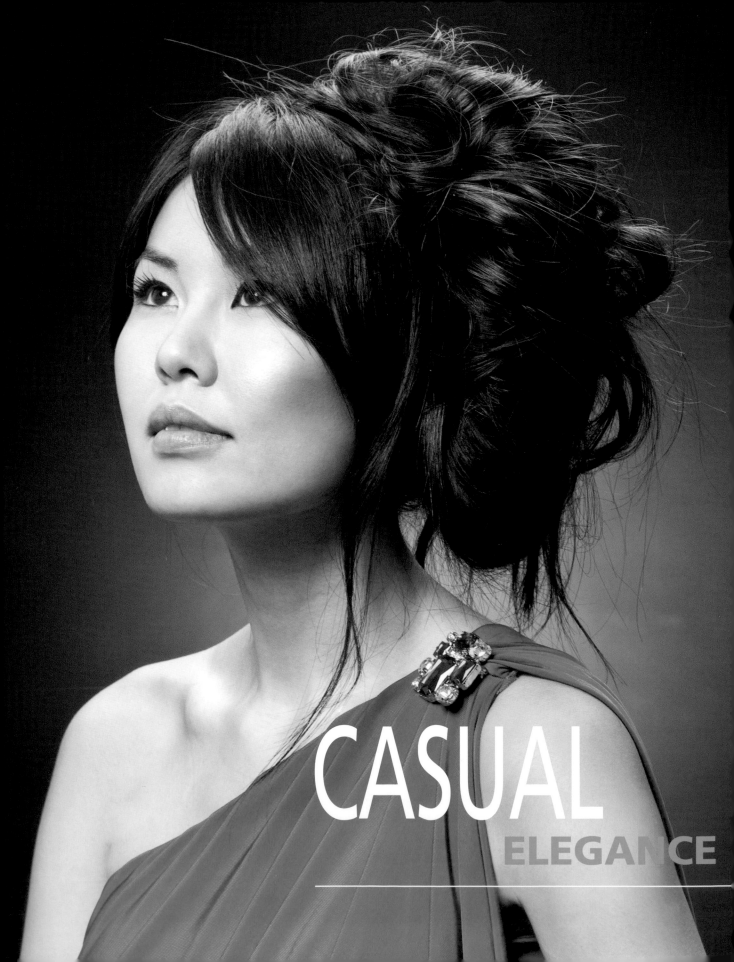

CASUAL
ELEGANCE

42

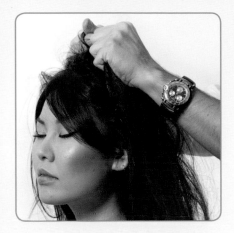

1. Wash and blow dry the hair. Rub in a bit of molding wax. Scrunch the hair with your hands for even application.

2. Be sure to apply wax throughout the hair, so that you can create the high style you want.

3. Gather the hair on one side of the head into a high ponytail.

4. Hold the ends of a section of hair in the ponytail, and backcomb the hair to the roots.

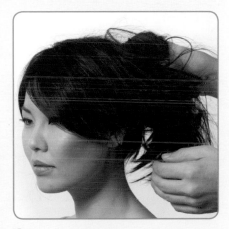

Loosely falling bangs create a natural front to this casually elegant look. The rest of the hair is folded into large, loose rings that are gathered in an arc at the top of the head.

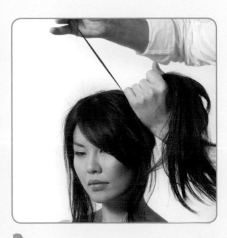

1

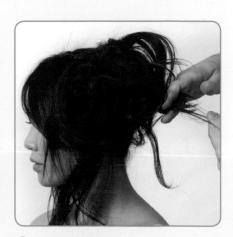

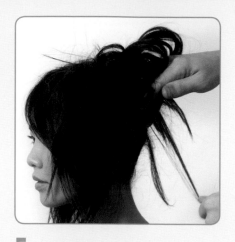

5

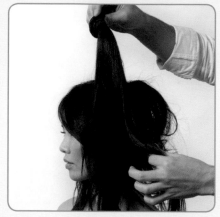

6

5. Repeat this process, backcombing all of the hair in the ponytail to create a natural, high volume ponytail.

6. Select a long hair extension that matches the color of the hair.

7. Secure the extension to the base of the ponytail with bobby pins.

8. Gather the hair and extension with your fingers and arrange them at the top of the head.

9. Once you are satisfied with the arrangement, secure the hairstyle with bobby pins.

10. Check the arrangement again, and make sure the style suits the shape of your face.

11. Add more bobby pins, as necessary, to keep the hair in place.

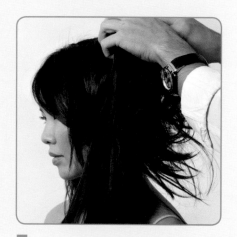

7

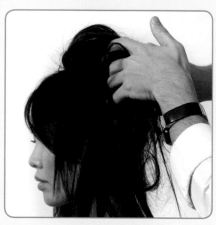

8

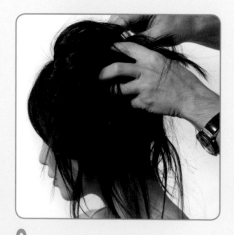

9

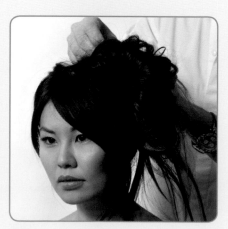

10

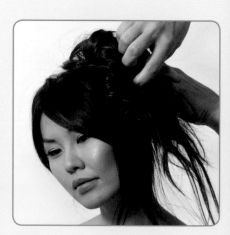

11

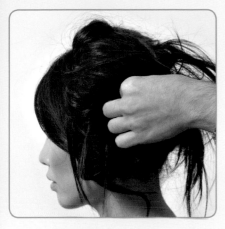

12

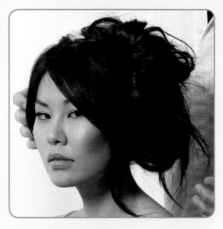

13

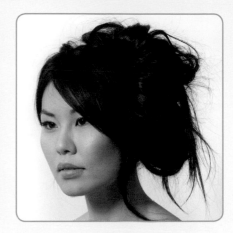

14

12. Gather the remaining loose hair randomly.

13. Draw some strands out of the arrangement so they hang loosely around the neck.

14. Mist the hair with holding spray.

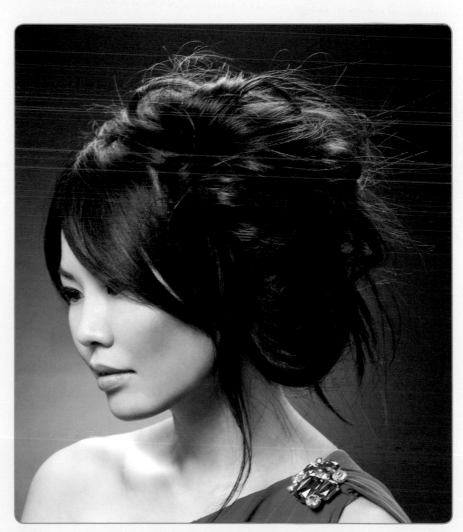

15

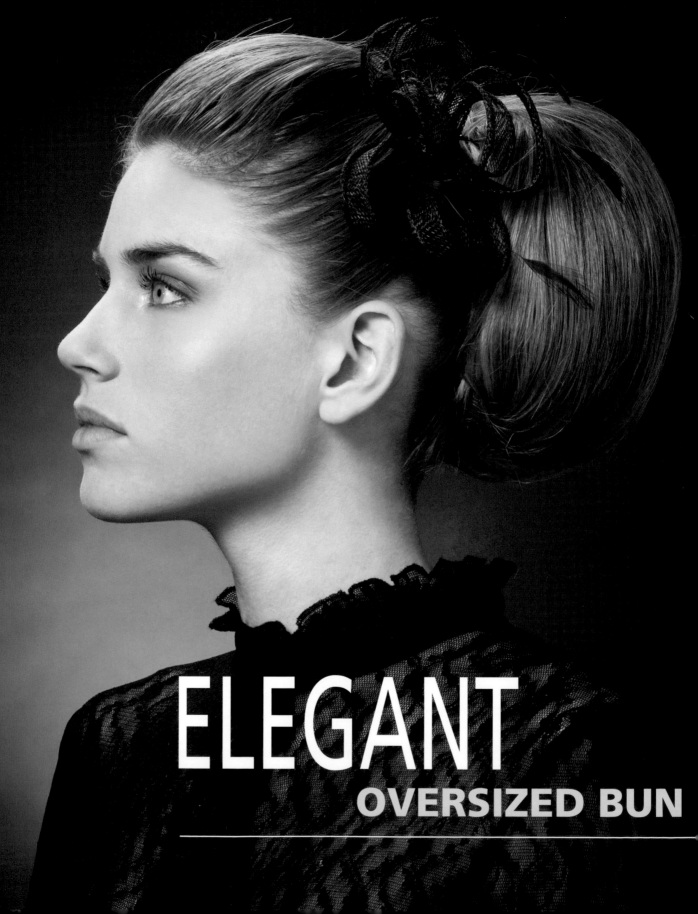

ELEGANT
OVERSIZED BUN

43

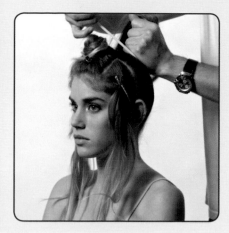

1

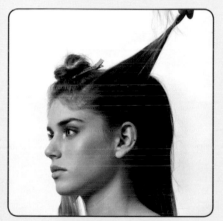

1. Wash and blow dry the hair. Make a part that extends from the top of each ear over the crown, and gather the hair below the part into a ponytail.

2. Divide the hair above the part into three sections, and secure each section with a clip.

3. Gather the middle section of hair at the front into a bun and secure at the top of the head. Brush back the hair on the right and left sides, mist with holding spray, and join with the ponytail at the back of the head.

4. Fold the ponytail forward over the crown and secure beside the bun at the top of the head.

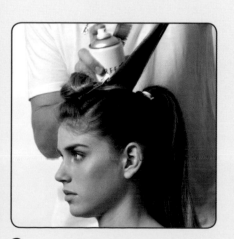

2

This clean and simple style features an oversized bun and smooth finish. If your natural hair is too short to cover the large bun, add hair extensions to the ponytail.

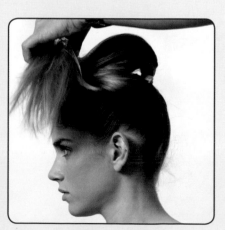

3

4

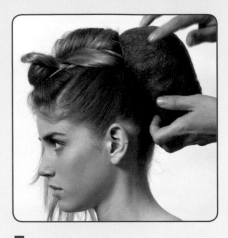

5

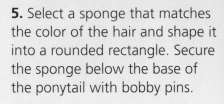
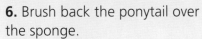
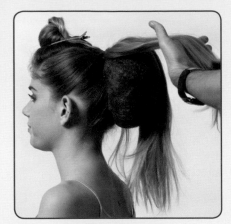

6

5. Select a sponge that matches the color of the hair and shape it into a rounded rectangle. Secure the sponge below the base of the ponytail with bobby pins.

6. Brush back the ponytail over the sponge.

7. Divide the hair in the ponytail into two sections and arrange the hair evenly over the sponge.

8. Comb one section of hair over the sponge. Secure the hair below the sponge, near the nape of the neck, with bobby pins.

9. Repeat with the other section of natural hair, and then mist the bun with holding spray.

10. Gather the hair ends and secure them under the sponge with bobby pins.

11. Check all around to make sure the ends are tucked under the ponytail.

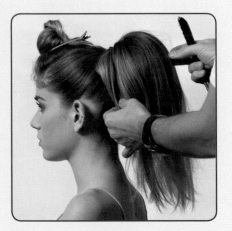

7

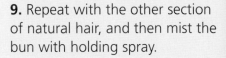
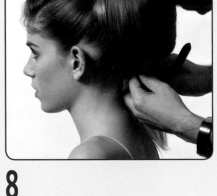

8

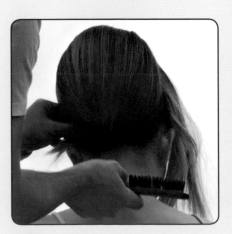

9

10

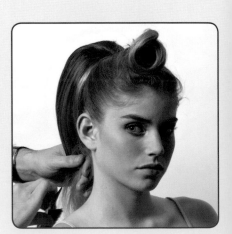

11

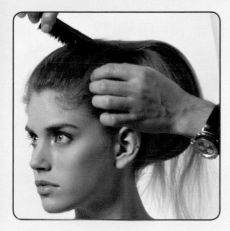

12

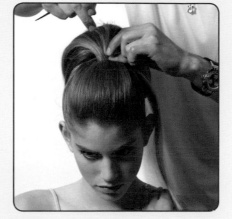

13

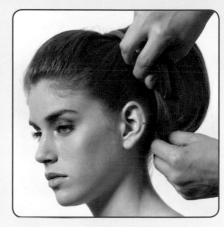

14

12. Release the bun at the top of the head and comb the hair backward.

13. Secure the hair near the top of the sponge with bobby pins.

14. Spread the hair from the front over the sponge, as before, and secure the ends underneath the sponge. Mist the hair with holding spray to secure.

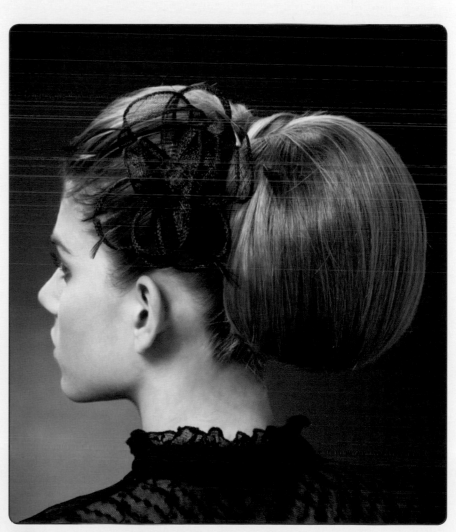

15

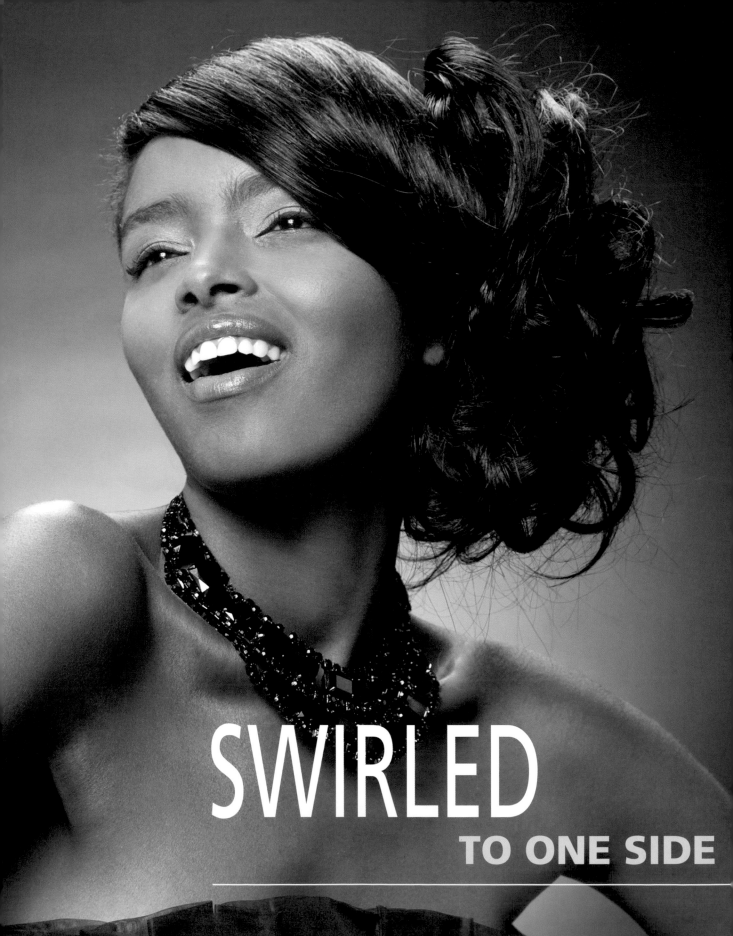

SWIRLED
TO ONE SIDE

44

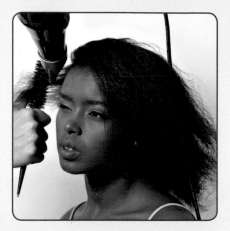

1

1. Wash and blow dry the hair straight.

2. Make a deep side part, and backcomb the overhanging hair. Select a long hair extension that matches the color of the hair.

3. Attach the extension to the hair just above the roots.

4. Extend a lock of hair from one side of the part to the other, and over the hair extension connection.

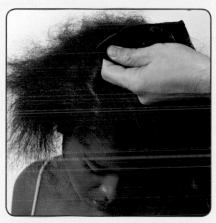

2

This dramatic hairstyle features a glorious collection of hair at one side of the head, exposing a seductively bare neck.

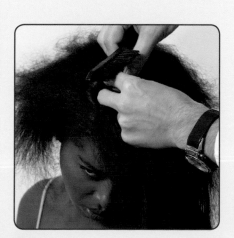

3

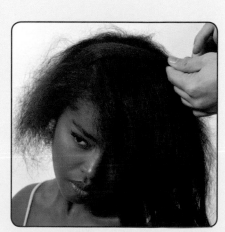

4

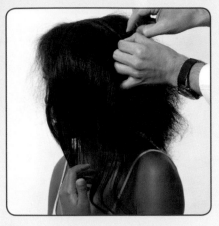

5

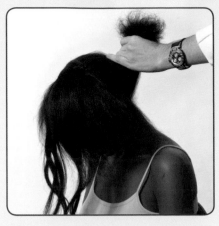

6

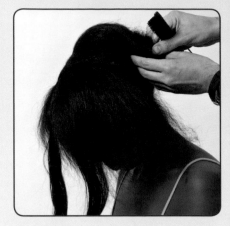

7

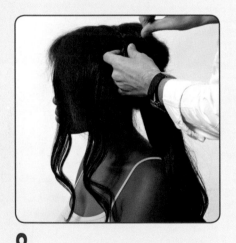

8

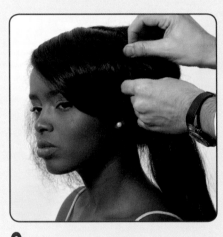

9

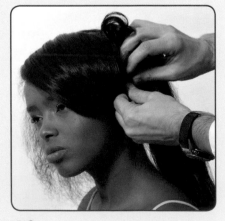

10

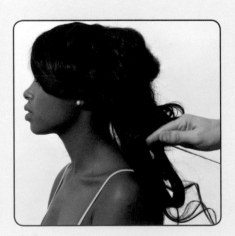

11

5. Affix the hair on the other side to conceal the point of connection.

6. Make a part that extends from behind each ear over the crown, and gather the hair below the part.

7. Make a sideway fold in the hair, and tuck in the roots. Secure the hair with bobby pins, making sure all the ends are tucked in.

8. Attach another long hair extension at the part line, on the same side as the first extension.

9. Gently comb the first extension backward, and tuck it behind the ear.

10. Secure the extension with bobby pins.

11. Hold a section of the extension by the ends, and backcomb the hair toward the root to add volume.

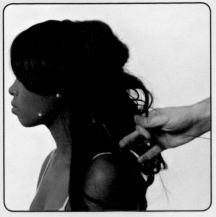

12

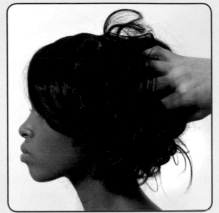

13

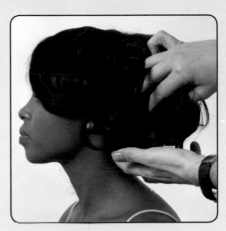

14

12. Repeat this process for all loose hair in the extension.

13. Gather the extension and lift it, shaping it in a loose and flowing manner.

14. Tuck the ends of the extension under the hair, and secure it with bobby pins. Mist with holding spray to finish.

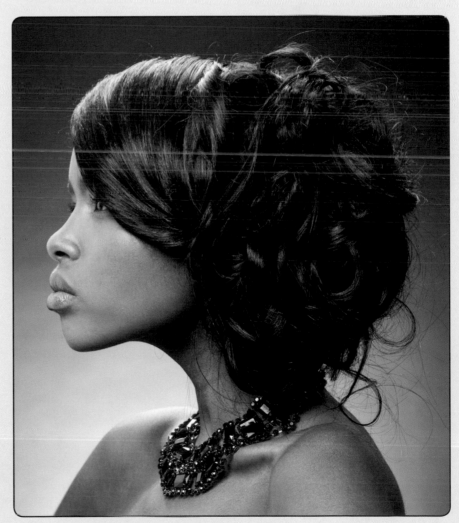

15

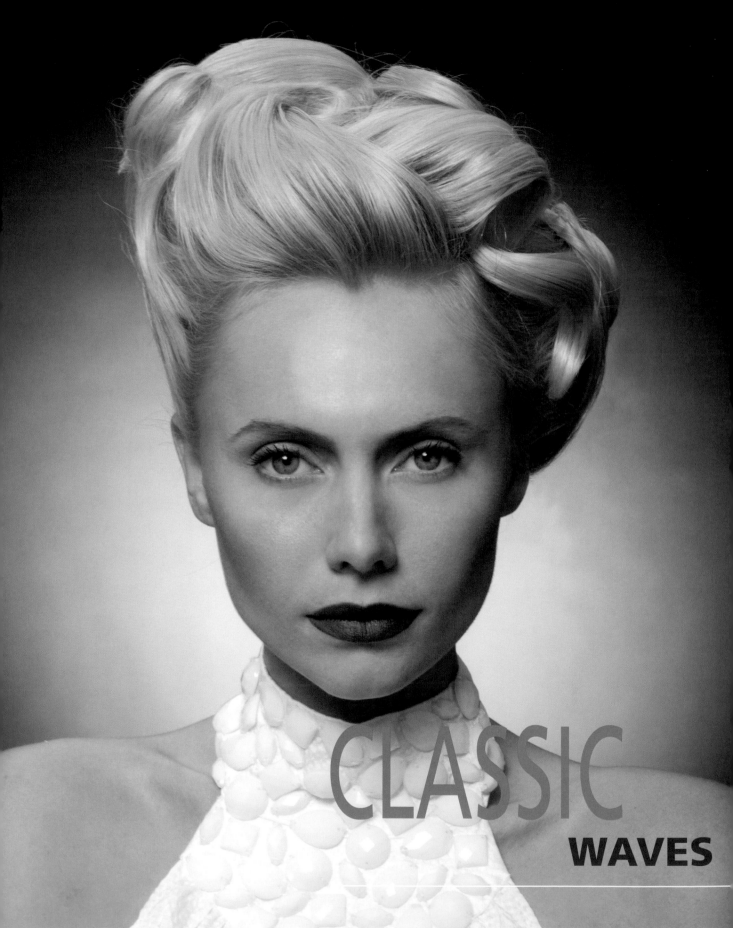

CLASSIC
WAVES

45

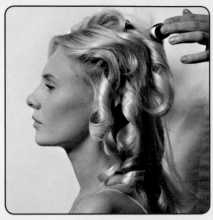

1

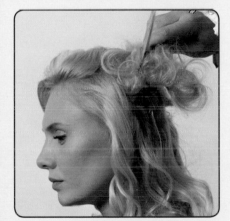

2

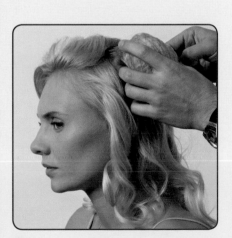

3

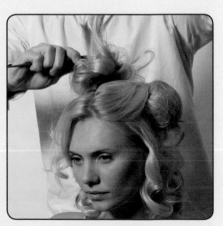

4

1. Wash and blow dry the hair. Separate the hair into 1-inch sections and curl each section into a loose ringlet with a medium curling iron.

2. Grasp the end of a ringlet near the back of the head, and backcomb it to the root.

3. Form a bun with the backcombed hair by wrapping it with a small hairnet. Select a hairnet color that contrasts with the hair color, for a textured look.

4. Grasp a curl near the middle of the head and backcomb it to the root. Form a bun with the backcombed hair.

In this hairstyle, the hair is swept away from the face in rich, luxurious waves. Reminiscent of Hollywood in the 1920s, the look is subtle and sensual.

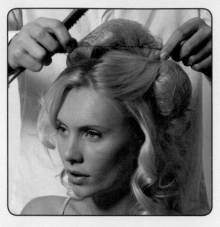

5

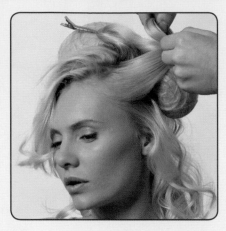

6

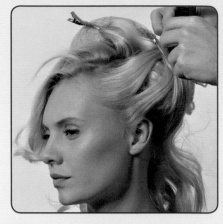

7

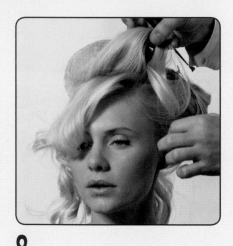

8

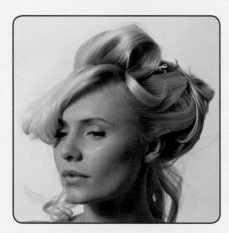

9

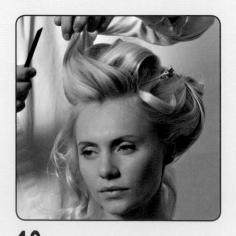

10

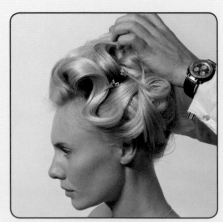

11

5. Wrap this section of hair with a small hairnet to make another bun, and secure it with a hairpin.

6. Brush back a section of hair at the front, and affix it with a bobby pin near the first bun.

7. Brush back another section of hair from the front, and affix it near the first bun.

8. Backcomb a section of hair near the brow, and draw it backward. Shape the hair into a high wave, and secure it near the crown of the head with a clip.

9. Mist the hair with holding spray to secure the shape. When hair is secure, remove the clip and insert bobby pins to secure.

10. Brush back the bangs while sculpting them upward, toward the crown of the head. Secure them near the top of the second bun. Continue to draw back sections of hair, shaping them to

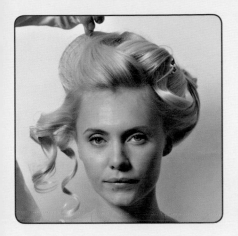

12

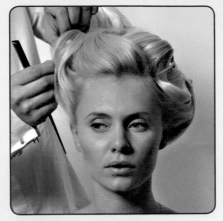

13

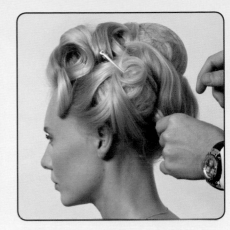

14

form high waves and securing each section to one of the two buns at the back of the head.

11. Mist each section of hair after drawing it backward, to secure it. Make sure to comb each section to create smooth waves.

12. Work your way gradually along the hairline, arranging the hair by sections and creating waves and swirls as you go.

13. Secure all the sections firmly, and mist them with holding spray.

14. Insert additional bobby pins and hair pins as needed, and mist the hair with holding spray. When the hair is secure, remove all clips.

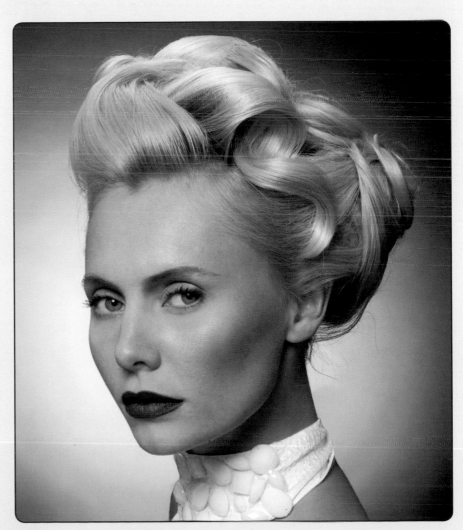

15

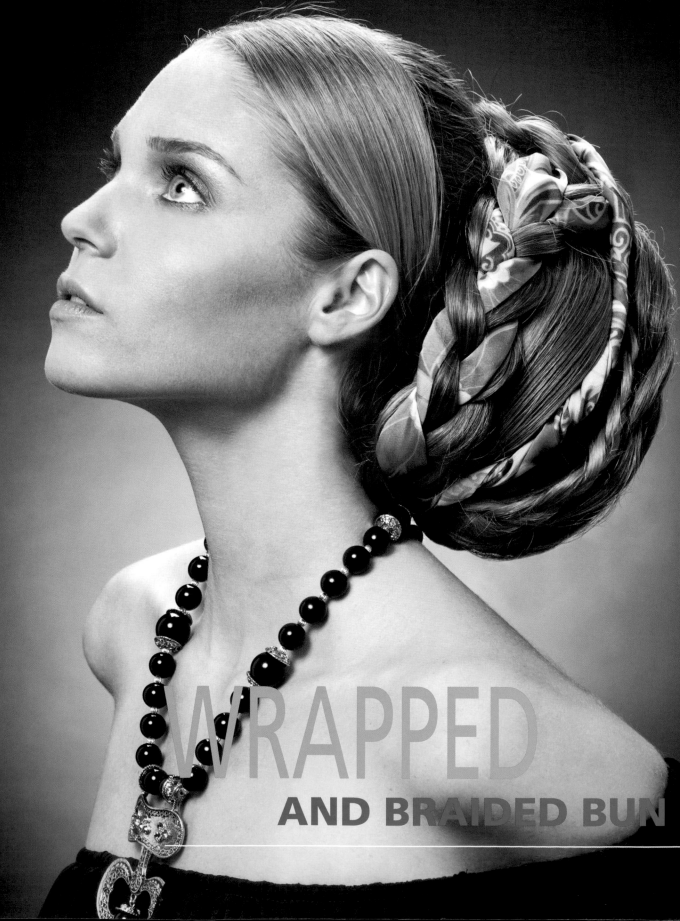

WRAPPED
AND BRAIDED BUN

46

Make the most of a couple of hair extensions by creating a large bun and long, braided rope. Integrate a couple of colorful ribbons to maximize the look.

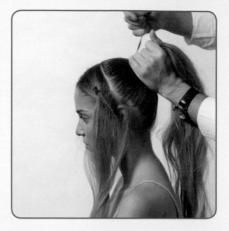

1

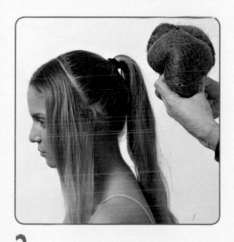

2

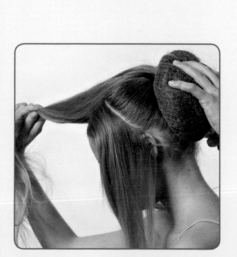

3

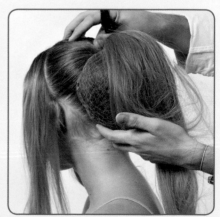

4

1. Wash and blow dry the hair. Make a part extending from the back of each ear and over the crown. Gather the hair below the part into a ponytail.

2. Select a sponge that matches the color of the hair, and shape it into a ball.

3. Bring the ponytail forward and attach the sponge to the back of the head, below the base of the ponytail, with bobby pins.

4. Bring the ponytail backward so that the hair falls over the top of the sponge.

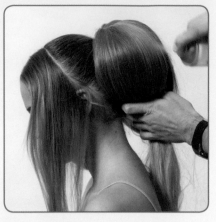

5

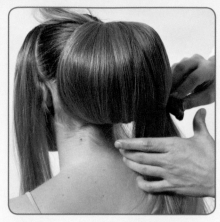

6

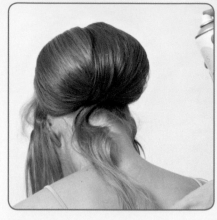

7

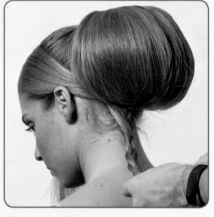

8

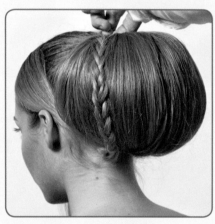

9

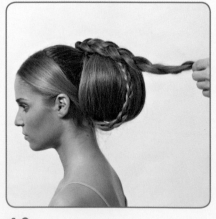

10

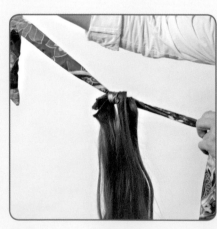

11

5. Separate the ponytail hair into two sections, and brush one section over the sponge. Secure the hair below the sponge with bobby pins, and mist it with holding spray to secure.

6. Brush out the other section of hair, and bring it over the sponge. Leave out a lock of hair for braiding later, and secure the rest below the sponge with bobby pins.

7. Mist the hair at the back of the head with holding spray to secure.

8. Brush the hair at the front of the head to one side, draw it to the back of the head, and braid it with the loose hair at the back of the head.

9. Fold the braid upward, bringing it up one side of the bun at the back of the head. Secure it at the top with bobby pins.

10. Select a hair extension that matches the color of the hair. Braid the extension and attach it

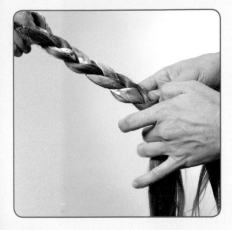

12

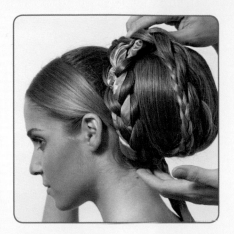

13

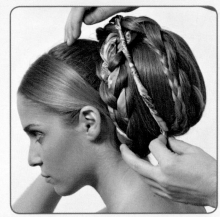

14

to the base of the ponytail, near the front, with bobby pins. Draw the braid over the bun, and secure it near the nape of the neck with bobby pins.

11. Select a hair extension that matches the color of the hair, and divide the extension into two sections. Tie a long, patterned ribbon to the middle of the extension, so that the ribbon hangs evenly on both sides.

12. Using both sections of the hair extension and one half of the ribbon, make a thick braid. Leave the other half of the ribbon loose.

13. Attach the braided extension at the top of the bun, and wrap it around one side of the bun, toward the nape of the neck. Affix it under the bun with bobby pins.

14. Wrap the loose end of the ribbon around itself and then around the bun. Affix it at the nape of the neck.

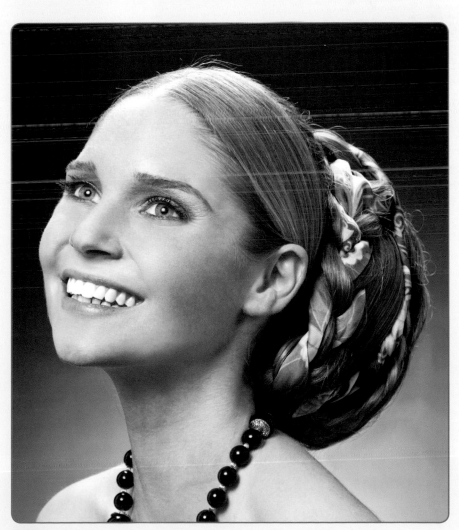

15

INDEX